WALL PLATE
FOR
SENIORS
OVER 60

The Essential Wall Plate Guide for Seniors

Tony D. Spaulding

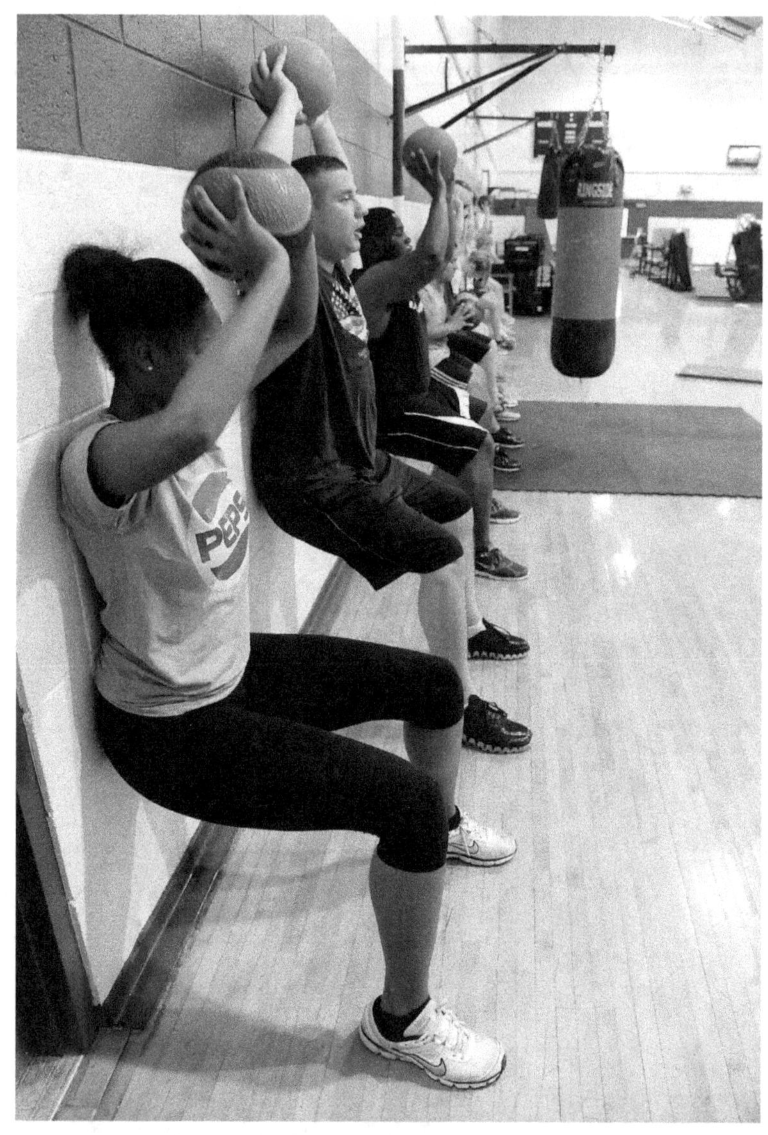

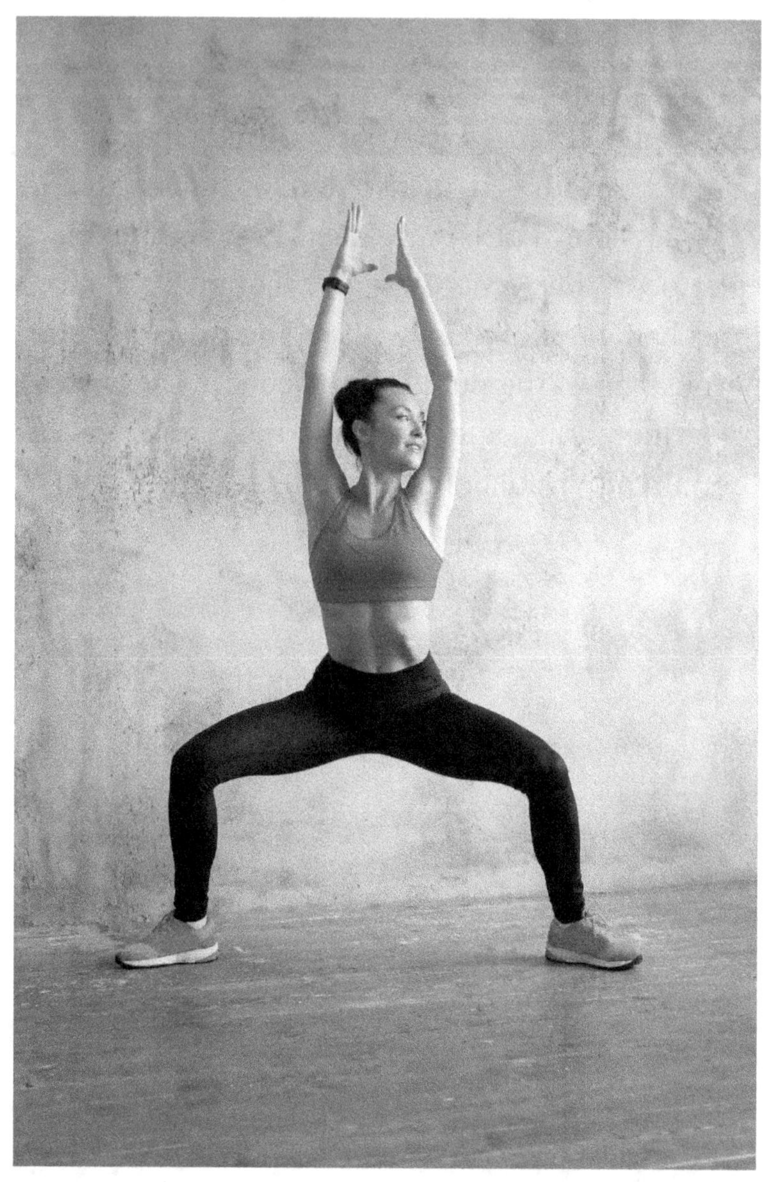

Table of Content

Conclusion

Conclusion

INTRODUCTION

Welcome to Wall Pilates for Seniors

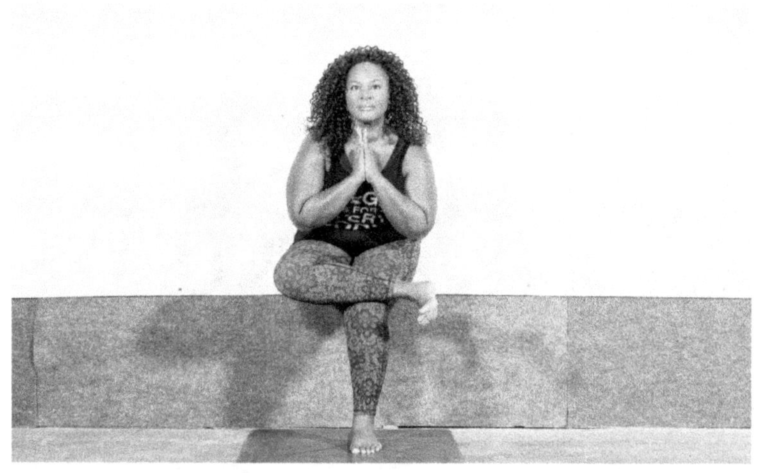

This Wall Pilates guide is designed to help seniors over 60 maintain strength, flexibility, and balance. As a certified Pilates coach, I'm thrilled to guide you through this transformative experience. Whether you're new to Pilates or looking to adapt your current routine, this book is your trusted companion for safe, effective exercises that meet you where you are.

Why Wall Pilates?

Wall Pilates offers the perfect blend of stability and support, making it ideal for seniors. The wall becomes your ally, helping you maintain proper alignment, reducing strain on your joints, and adding an extra layer of safety as you move through various exercises. This gentle yet powerful form of Pilates can improve your core strength, enhance mobility, and boost your confidence in everyday activities.

Benefits of Wall Pilates

1. As we age, maintaining balance becomes crucial to prevent falls and maintain independence. Wall Pilates focuses on strengthening the muscles that support balance—your core, legs, and back. The wall provides a stable surface to lean on or press against, giving you the confidence to push yourself safely.

2. One of the key principles of Pilates is controlled, flowing movements that reduce stress on your joints. With Wall Pilates, you can gently stretch and strengthen muscles without overextending or risking injury. This is particularly beneficial if you're dealing with conditions like arthritis or joint stiffness.

3. Wall Pilates helps correct your alignment by encouraging proper posture in each exercise. Over time, you'll stand taller, sit straighter, and move more freely.

4. You don't need to lift heavy weights or engage in intense workouts to build strength. Wall Pilates uses your body's resistance, along with the support of the wall, to tone muscles safely and effectively. Each exercise can be adapted to your current fitness level, allowing you to progress at your own pace.

As your coach, I want you to know that Wall Pilates is for everyone—whether you're completely new to exercise or have been active for years. The key is to start slow and listen to your body. Pilates is not about perfection; it's about progress. With consistent practice, even 10-15 minutes a day, you'll notice improvements in how you move, feel and carry yourself.

What to Expect

In the following chapters, we'll explore a variety of Wall Pilates exercises that focus on different aspects of your health. You'll begin with simple movements, like wall-supported squats and stretches, designed to warm up your muscles and get you comfortable using the wall for support. As you progress, we'll introduce more challenging exercises that strengthen your core, legs, and arms, always with modifications to suit your needs.

Each exercise includes clear instructions, safety tips, and variations so you can make adjustments based on how your body feels each day. Remember, Pilates is a journey, and the wall is your guide.

How to Use This Book

The first few chapters introduce you to the fundamentals of Pilates and the specific benefits of Wall Pilates for seniors. If you're new to Pilates or haven't exercised in a while, I recommend starting here to build a strong foundation. Even if you're familiar with exercise, these chapters will help you understand how to use the wall for proper alignment and support.

This book is divided into sections that gradually increase in difficulty. Begin with the Basic Exercises section to familiarize yourself with movements that are gentle but effective. Once you're comfortable, move on to the Intermediate and Advanced exercises when you feel ready. Each exercise includes step-by-step instructions and tips to ensure you're performing the movements safely and correctly. Everyone's body is different, and your workout should reflect that. The Customizing Your Workout section will show you how to create routines that cater to your specific goals and abilities. Whether you want to focus on balance, strength, or flexibility, this book offers a variety of exercises to suit your needs. You'll also find ways to modify exercises to make them easier or more challenging, depending on how you feel that day. For every exercise, you'll find easy-to-follow diagrams and clear descriptions to guide you. You'll also see coaching tips scattered throughout the book to remind you of the little things like keeping your core engaged or breathing steadily during each move. These tips are designed to make your practice more enjoyable and effective. There's no rush. Pilates is a practice of control and precision, not speed. You may find that some exercises feel easier than others, and that's perfectly fine. Listen to your body and take breaks when needed. Move through the book at a pace that feels right for you. If you're feeling strong, you can challenge yourself with new exercises. If you need a gentler approach, stick with the basics until you're ready to progress.

If you're dealing with specific health concerns like arthritis, osteoporosis, or balance issues, the

Special Considerations for Seniors section is where you'll find modifications tailored to your condition. Pilates can be incredibly supportive for managing chronic conditions, and this book ensures that you're practicing in a way that's safe and beneficial. Pilates isn't just about the exercises you do on the mat or at the wall. The Incorporating Wall Pilates into Daily Life chapter helps you integrate these movements into your routine, so you can stay active throughout the day. Whether it's simple stretches while standing or using the wall to improve posture while sitting, this section provides tips to make Pilates a natural part of your daily life.

Improvement in Pilates often happens in small, noticeable ways—like standing taller, moving more comfortably, or feeling more balanced. Throughout the book, I encourage you to keep track of how you're feeling as you practice. By following the recommended routines and progressing slowly, you'll see improvements in strength, flexibility, and overall well-being over time. It's important to remember that consistency is key. Even if you only practice a few exercises a day, you'll build strength and improve mobility over time. The Frequently Asked Questions section will help answer any concerns or questions you may have as you progress. And when you need a little inspiration, the Success Stories chapter offers real-life examples of seniors just like you who have transformed their lives through Wall Pilates.

This book is your guide to becoming more confident in your movements and enhancing your quality of life. Every page is designed to support your journey to better health, offering simple steps to help you feel stronger, move with ease, and improve your overall well-being.

Now it's time to take the first step. Find a sturdy wall, take a deep breath, and let's begin this exciting journey together!

CHAPTER 1

Understanding Wall Pilates

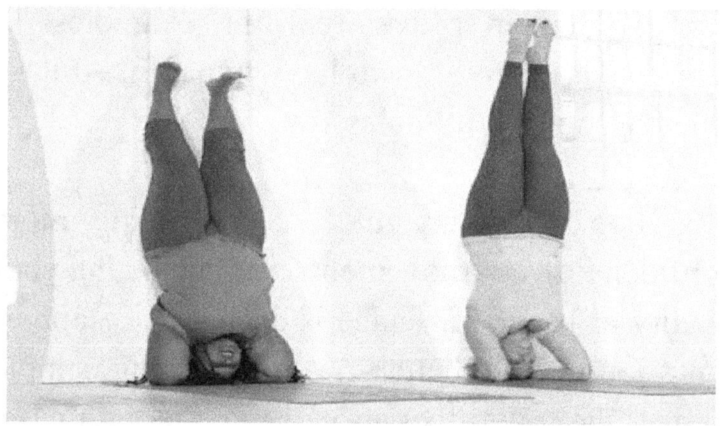

Wall Pilates is not just another workout—it's a gentle, effective way to build strength, improve flexibility, and boost your balance, all while using the wall as your partner. Let's break down what Wall Pilates is, why it's so beneficial for seniors, and how you can get the most out of your practice.

What is Wall Pilates?

Wall Pilates is a variation of traditional Pilates that uses the wall for support, stability, and alignment. In a typical Pilates class, many movements happen on a mat or using specialized equipment, but Wall Pilates focuses on making the exercises more accessible by incorporating a sturdy surface—your wall. This added support makes it easier to maintain balance and proper form, which is especially important as we age.

Here's why Wall Pilates stands out:

1. The wall provides a solid foundation, allowing you to engage your muscles safely without the fear of falling.
2. It helps guide your movements, ensuring that your posture is aligned and your form is correct.
3. The resistance of your body weight against the wall strengthens muscles without putting stress on your joints.

The Principles of Pilates for Seniors

Pilates is built on six core principles, and Wall Pilates follows these same guidelines to promote a well-rounded approach to fitness. Let's take a look at these principles and how they apply to your practice:

1. Pilates is a mindful exercise. It requires focus on each movement to ensure you're engaging the right muscles and maintaining proper form. When using the wall, you'll concentrate on how your body moves in relation to the wall, which enhances awareness of your posture and alignment.

2. Every movement in Pilates is intentional and controlled. Wall Pilates allows you to work at your own pace, with the wall providing the necessary support to perform each exercise with precision. This control helps prevent injury and makes the exercises more effective.

3. Pilates is all about engaging your core— the muscles around your abdomen, lower

back, and pelvis. This area, often referred to as your "powerhouse," supports every movement. In Wall Pilates, you'll frequently engage your core while the wall provides balance and stability, making it easier to focus on strengthening this crucial area.

4. Pilates movements are smooth and continuous, never rushed. With Wall Pilates, the wall acts as a guide to help you transition between exercises seamlessly, ensuring that your movements remain fluid and graceful.

5. Every movement in Pilates has a purpose, and the goal is to execute each exercise with perfect form. The wall helps you maintain this precision, especially when you're learning new exercises. You'll be able to focus on the quality of your movements, not just the quantity.

6. In Pilates, breath is coordinated with movement to help you stay focused and relaxed. Breathing deeply and consistently while using the wall allows you to get the

most out of each exercise, improving circulation and reducing tension.

Why Wall Pilates is Perfect for Seniors

As we age, our bodies change. Joints may become stiffer, balance can become more challenging, and we may not have the same strength or flexibility we once had. Wall Pilates addresses these changes in a way that is supportive and empowering. Here's why it's a fantastic choice for seniors:

1. Wall Pilates offers low-impact exercises that are easy on your joints. The support from the wall allows you to engage muscles without putting strain on your knees, hips, or lower back, making it an ideal option if you have arthritis or other joint issues.

2. It Improves Balance and Coordination. As we get older, balance can become a concern, but Wall Pilates helps you strengthen the muscles that stabilize your body. The wall provides an added layer of

safety, so you can focus on improving your balance without fear of falling.

3. It Increases Flexibility. One of the key benefits of Pilates is improving flexibility. Using the wall allows you to stretch deeper while maintaining control, which can be particularly beneficial if you feel stiff or tight in certain areas.

4. It Strengthens Core and Posture. Good posture is essential for maintaining mobility and preventing back pain. Wall Pilates focuses on core strength, which is the foundation of good posture. You'll also be using the wall to align your spine and shoulders correctly, helping you stand taller and feel more confident in your movements.

5. One of the best things about Wall Pilates is that it's adaptable. Whether you're just starting out or have been active for years, you can modify each exercise to suit your fitness level. The wall allows you to adjust the intensity of your movements, so you

can progress at a pace that's comfortable for you.

Safety Considerations

Your safety is always my top priority. While Wall Pilates is generally very safe, there are a few key points to keep in mind:

1. If something doesn't feel right, don't push yourself. Take breaks as needed and modify exercises to fit your comfort level.
2. Make sure the wall you're using is strong and flat, without any obstructions. A smooth, stable surface will help you perform the exercises safely.
3. Rushing through exercises can lead to improper form and increase the risk of injury. Focus on slow, deliberate movements and breathe consistently.
4. Even though Pilates is a low-impact workout, it's important to stay hydrated, especially during longer sessions.

How Wall Pilates Helps in Daily Life

The beauty of Wall Pilates is that the benefits extend far beyond your workout. As you improve your strength, flexibility, and balance, you'll notice positive changes in your daily life:

1. You'll be able to **move more comfortably** throughout the day, whether you're getting up from a chair, reaching for something on a shelf, or climbing stairs.
2. Your posture will improve, helping to alleviate **back or neck pain** and allowing you to stand tall with confidence.
3. You'll gain more control over your **balance**, reducing your risk of falls and making everyday activities safer and easier.

Now that you understand the principles and benefits of **Wall Pilates**, it's time to start moving! Each exercise in this book is designed to build on what you've learned here, helping you gain strength, mobility, and confidence with every session.

CHAPTER 2

Getting Started

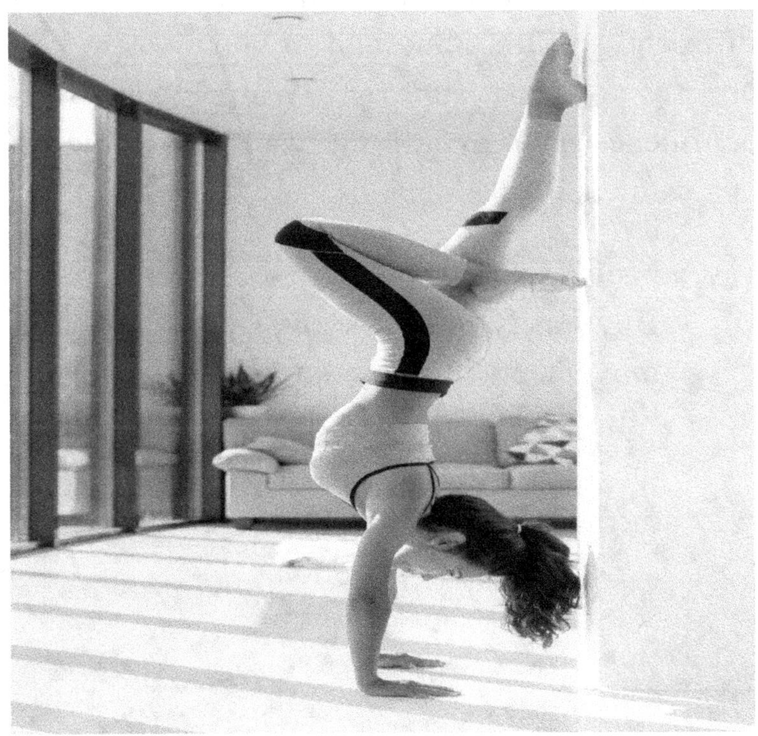

Before we start moving, it's important to assess your current fitness level, gather the right equipment, set up your space, and warm up properly. By preparing in this way, you'll ensure that your practice is both safe and effective. Let's get started!

Before you begin, take a moment to assess how your body feels today. Everyone's fitness level is different, and it's important to know where you are so you can approach Wall Pilates with confidence and avoid injury. Here's how to evaluate your fitness level:

1. **Mobility**

   How easily can you move? Try some basic movements like standing up from a chair, lifting your arms overhead, or bending at the knees. If any of these motions feel difficult or cause discomfort, note which areas need extra attention.

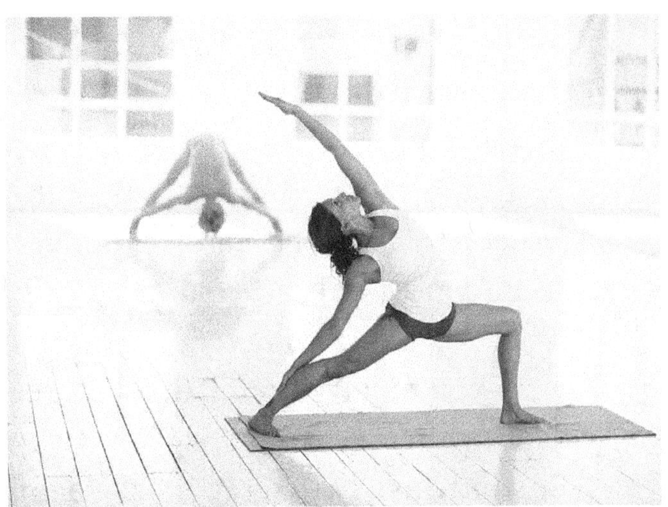

2. Balance

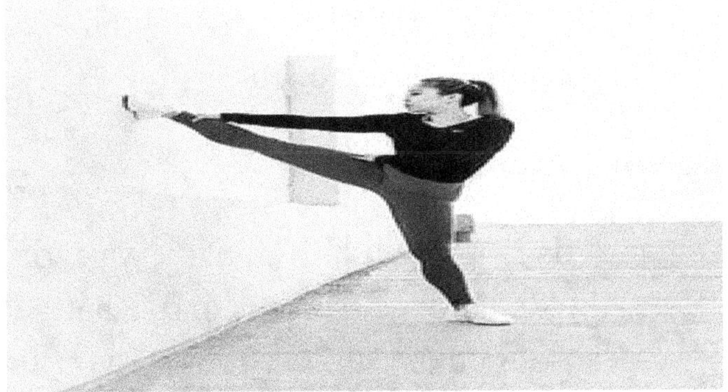

Balance is key to many Pilates exercises. Stand near a wall and see if you can lift one foot off the ground while maintaining stability. If balance is a challenge, don't worry! Wall Pilates is specifically designed to improve this.

3. **Strength**

   Consider your current strength level, especially in your core, legs, and arms. You don't need to be strong to start Wall Pilates, but knowing where you stand will help you modify exercises when needed.

4. **Endurance**

   If you're used to short bursts of activity but feel fatigued quickly, that's okay. Pilates is all about slow, controlled movements, so it's important to listen to your body and take breaks as needed.

Keep in Mind:

- This is not a test! It's just a way for you to understand your body and what it needs. Throughout this book, you'll find modifications for each exercise to match your current fitness level and help you progress over time.

Essential Equipment and Gear

To get the most out of your **Wall Pilates** practice, you'll need a few simple items to ensure you're comfortable, supported, and set up for success. The beauty of Wall Pilates is that it doesn't require any complicated or expensive equipment, but the right gear can make a significant difference in your experience and progress.

Here's a breakdown of the essentials you'll need to begin:

1. A Sturdy Wall

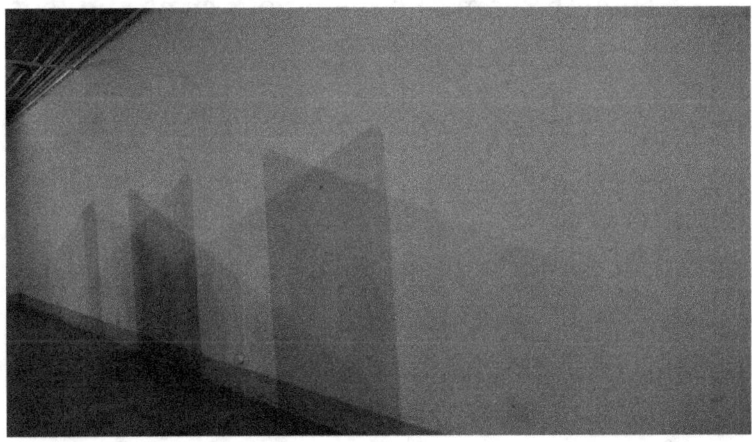

The **wall** is the foundation of your practice. It provides the stability and support you'll rely on during exercises. When selecting the right wall, keep these factors in mind:

1. Make sure the wall is flat and smooth without any obstacles like picture frames, switches, or shelves. A clear wall helps you move freely and maintain correct posture.
2. Choose a wall that's solid and reliable. Avoid areas with doors or windows nearby where there could be distractions or instability.
3. You should have at least a few feet of space around you to move comfortably, with enough room to stretch your arms and legs without feeling cramped.

2. Comfortable Clothing

Wearing the right clothing is essential for unrestricted movement and comfort. Choose clothing that's breathable, stretchy, and not too loose to ensure you can move easily without any fabric getting in the way.

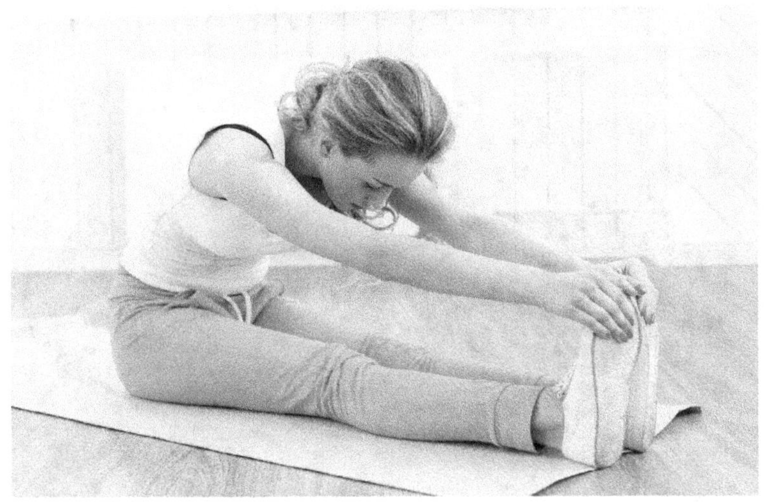

1. Form-fitting attire like leggings, yoga pants, or stretchable shorts paired with a fitted top is ideal for Pilates.
2. Since Pilates involves slow, controlled movements, you may not get overheated quickly, but layering with a light jacket or sweater that you can remove as you warm up can be useful.
3. Avoid bulky items like sweatpants or oversized shirts, which may interfere with your movements or make it difficult to see how your body is aligned.

3. Supportive Footwear or Barefoot

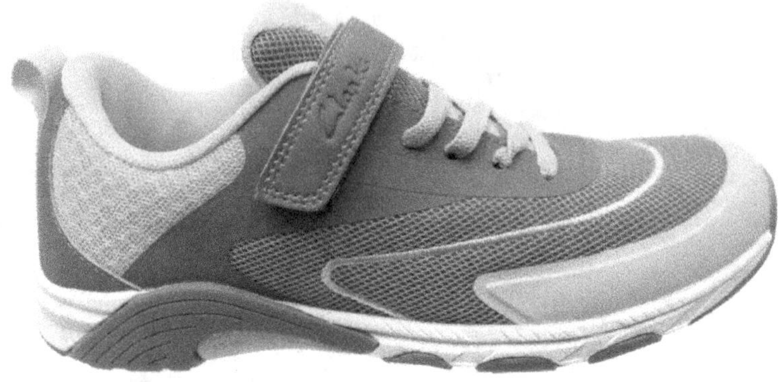

Footwear is a personal choice in Wall Pilates, and it's all about what makes you feel most comfortable and secure:

1. **Barefoot**: Many people practice Pilates barefoot to help with balance, feel the floor more fully, and engage their foot muscles more effectively. Going barefoot can help you stay grounded and improve your stability.

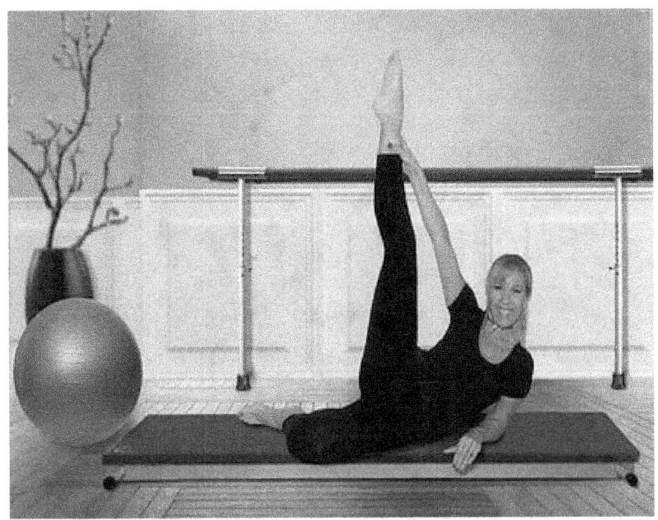

2. **Grippy Socks**: If you prefer to wear something on your feet, choose Pilates or yoga socks that have non-slip grips on the bottom. These help prevent slipping while allowing you to stay flexible and connected to the ground.

3. **Supportive Shoes**: If you have sensitive feet or prefer more stability, lightweight sneakers or supportive athletic shoes can be worn. Choose shoes that are flexible, yet supportive enough to allow for full range of motion in your feet and ankles.

4. Mat (Optional)

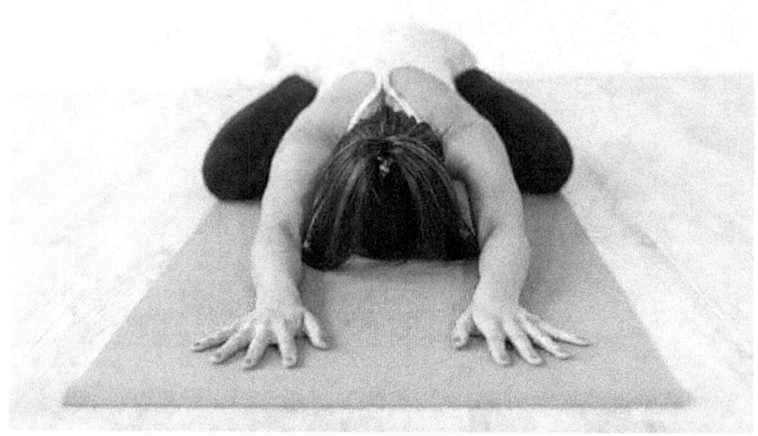

A **mat** can add extra comfort to your practice, particularly if you'll be standing for long periods or if you occasionally need to sit or kneel for certain exercises. Here's why a mat might be useful:

1. **Joint Cushioning**: If you have sensitive knees, hips, or feet, a soft mat can provide some cushioning and prevent discomfort on hard floors.
2. **Traction**: A non-slip mat can help prevent slipping, especially if you're barefoot or wearing socks.

3. **Stability**: A mat can create a designated space for your workout, helping you stay centered and focused on your movements without worrying about sliding or losing your balance.

5. Chair (Optional)

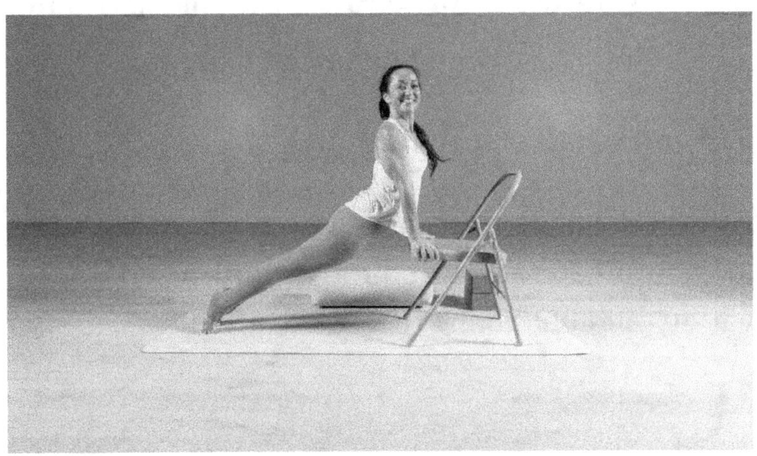

If you're just starting out or have limited mobility, having a **chair** nearby can provide additional support and help you modify certain exercises.

1. A sturdy chair with a back can act as an extension of the wall to help you keep your

balance, particularly for exercises that involve standing on one leg or shifting your weight.

2. Some exercises may call for seated modifications, especially if you have difficulty standing for long periods. A chair can give you the option to complete exercises while sitting, without sacrificing form or effectiveness.

6. Pilates Ball (Optional)

As you advance in your practice, you might want to incorporate a **small Pilates ball** to add more variety and challenge to your workouts.

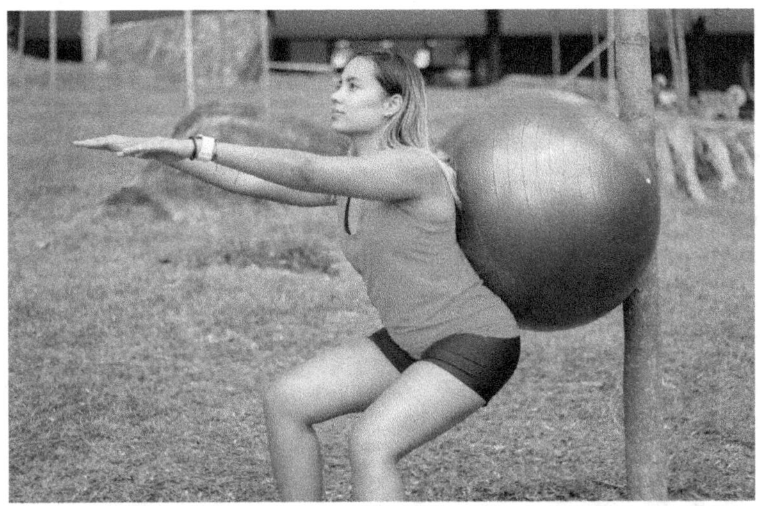

1. Holding the ball between your hands or legs during certain exercises can increase engagement of your core muscles.
2. Using the ball in conjunction with the wall can provide an extra challenge for balance-based exercises, helping to build stability in your core and legs.
3. The ball can be used to assist in stretches or provide gentle resistance during certain movements, adding versatility to your practice.

7. Water Bottle and Towel

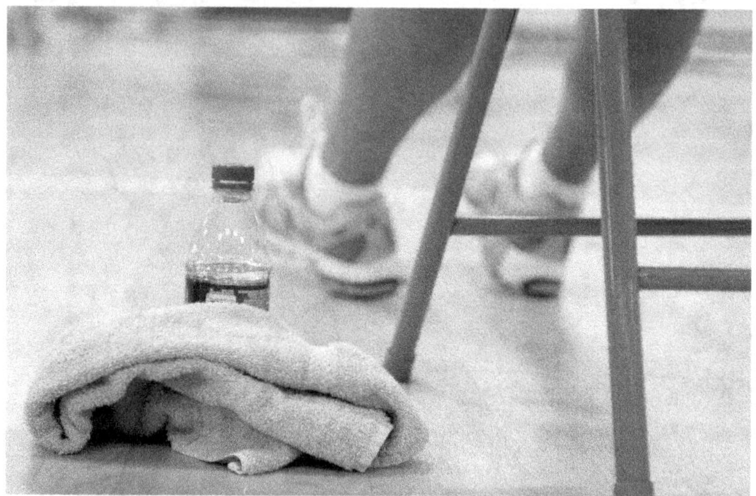

While **Wall Pilates** is a low-impact form of exercise, it's still important to stay hydrated throughout your session, especially if you're working through several exercises in succession.

1. Keep a **water bottle** nearby and take small sips during breaks to stay refreshed.
2. A **towel** can also come in handy to wipe away sweat or to add a little extra padding if needed on sensitive joints.

Why Proper Gear Matters

Each of these items is selected to enhance your **Wall Pilates** experience. By preparing yourself with the right equipment, you ensure:

1. The wall provides the necessary stability and support to maintain proper posture and alignment, reducing the risk of injury.
2. Wearing appropriate clothing and footwear keeps you comfortable, while a mat or chair can add extra cushioning or support when needed.
3. With your gear and space set up, you'll be able to focus entirely on your movements, allowing you to perform each exercise with precision and control.

By taking a few moments to prepare with the right equipment and gear, you set the foundation for a safe, effective, and enjoyable **Wall Pilates** session.

Setting Up Your Space

Creating the right environment for your Pilates practice is essential for success. You don't need a fancy studio—just a quiet, clear space with enough room to move comfortably.

1. Ensure that the wall you'll be using is clear of any furniture, artwork, or other objects that could interfere with your movements. You'll need about a foot or two of space between yourself and the wall for most exercises.
2. Make sure the room is well-lit so you can see your movements and maintain focus during each exercise.
3. Choose a space where you won't be distracted. Pilates is a mindful practice, and having a calm environment will help you concentrate on your body and your breath.
4. You may prefer to practice in silence, allowing you to focus entirely on your breathing and movements. Alternatively, some light, relaxing music can enhance your experience, helping you maintain a

steady rhythm as you flow through the exercises.

Warm-Up Exercises

Warming up is a critical part of any workout, especially for seniors. A good warm-up gets your blood flowing, loosens your joints, and prepares your muscles for movement. Here are a few gentle warm-up exercises to get you ready for your Wall Pilates session:

1. Wall Shoulder Rolls

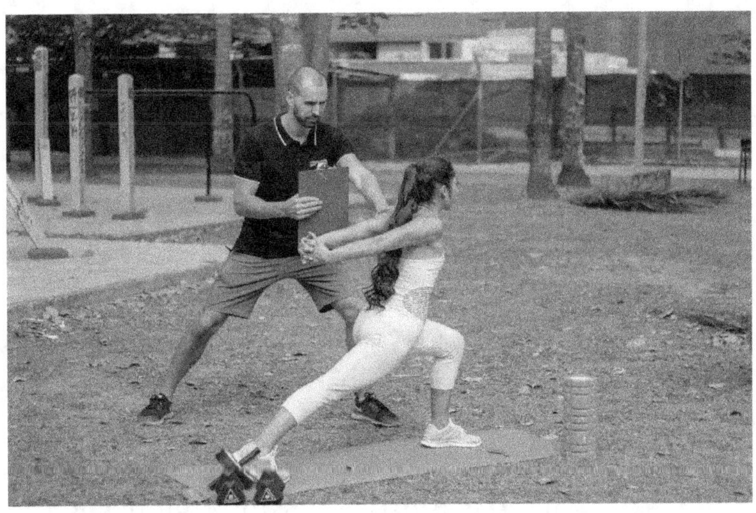

a. Stand with your back gently pressed against the wall.

b. Roll your shoulders forward in a circular motion, bringing them up towards your ears and then down.

c. Repeat 5 times, then reverse the motion.

d. This helps loosen tight shoulder muscles and improve your posture.

2. Wall Marching

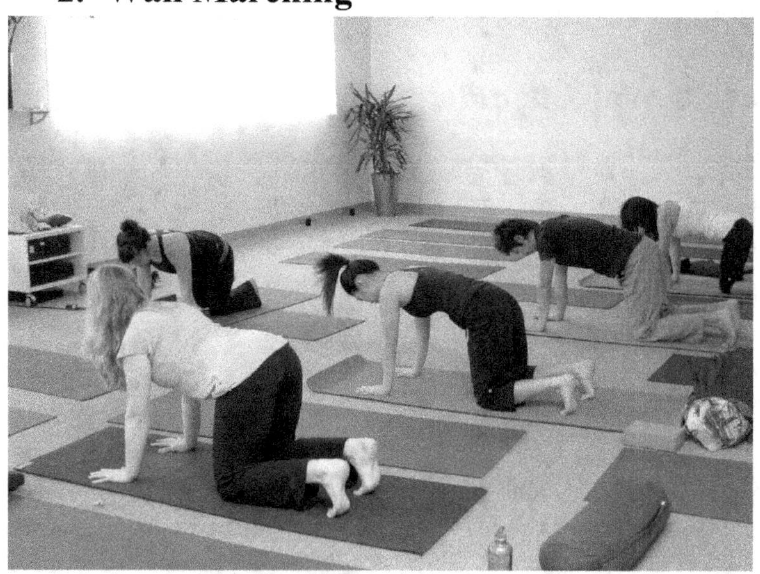

a. Stand facing the wall, with your hands lightly pressing against it for support.

b. Slowly lift one knee toward your chest, as if you're marching in place, then lower it back down.

c. Alternate legs and repeat 10-12 times on each side.

d. This warms up your hips, legs, and core, while gently increasing your heart rate.

3. Standing Heel Raises

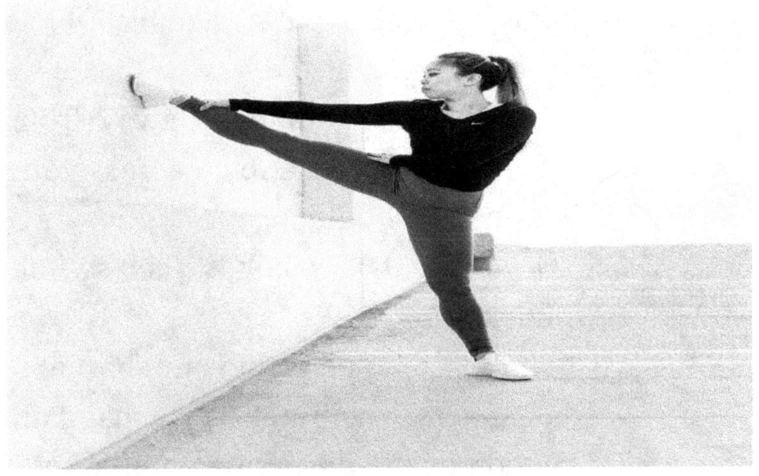

a. Stand facing the wall with your hands resting on it for balance.

b. Slowly rise up onto the balls of your feet, lifting your heels off the ground, then lower back down.

c. Repeat 10 times.

d. This exercise wakes up your calf muscles and strengthens your ankles, improving stability.

4. Wall Chest Stretch

a. Stand facing the side of the wall, placing your palm against it at shoulder height.

b. Gently twist your body away from the wall to feel a stretch across your chest and shoulders.

c. Hold for 10-15 seconds, then switch sides.

d. This stretch opens up your chest and shoulders, helping you maintain good posture during your exercises.

Now that you've assessed your fitness level, gathered your equipment, set up your space, and completed a gentle warm-up, you're ready to begin your Wall Pilates practice! Remember, take your time, listen to your body, and focus on steady, controlled movements. This is your time to strengthen and rejuvenate, one step at a time.

CHAPTER 3

Basic Wall Pilates Exercises

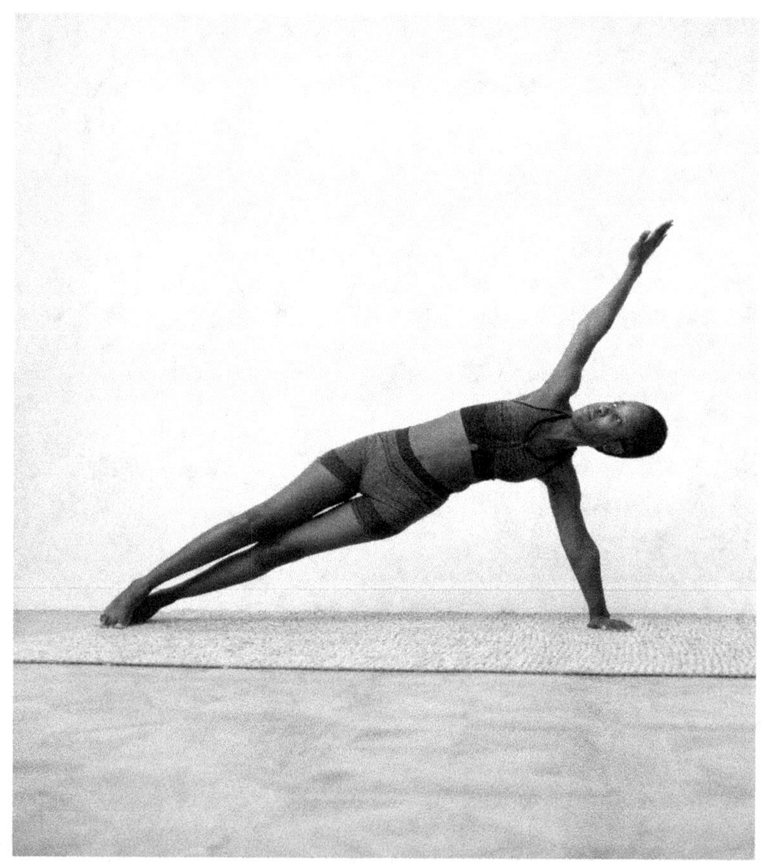

These exercises are specifically designed with seniors in mind, using the wall to support and stabilize you as you move. Whether you're just starting your Pilates journey or have some experience, these foundational exercises will help you build confidence while improving your body's mobility.

Each exercise is meant to be performed slowly and mindfully, focusing on breathing, alignment, and control. Let's begin!

Introduction to Basic Exercises

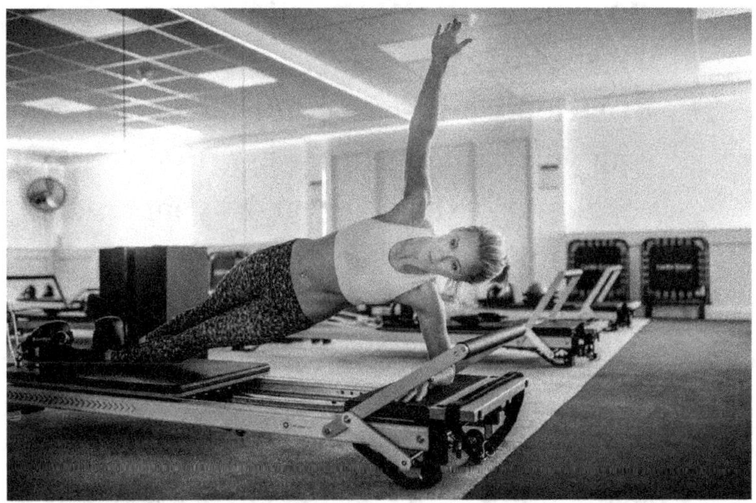

These basic exercises are perfect for getting accustomed to the benefits of **Wall Pilates**. The wall serves as your anchor, offering stability and support for movements that improve core strength, posture, and overall flexibility. Each of the following exercises is low-impact, so they're gentle on your joints while still providing an effective workout.

Key Points to Remember:

- **Move at Your Own Pace**: There's no rush. Focus on smooth, controlled movements. Pilates is all about precision, not speed.
- **Breathing**: Always coordinate your breath with your movements. Inhale through your nose and exhale through your mouth, staying mindful of each breath.
- **Alignment**: Pay attention to your posture, keeping your spine straight and core engaged.
- **Modifications**: If an exercise feels too challenging, don't hesitate to use a chair for

extra support or reduce the range of motion. Always listen to your body.

Now, let's break down each exercise step by step.

Exercise 1: Wall Squats

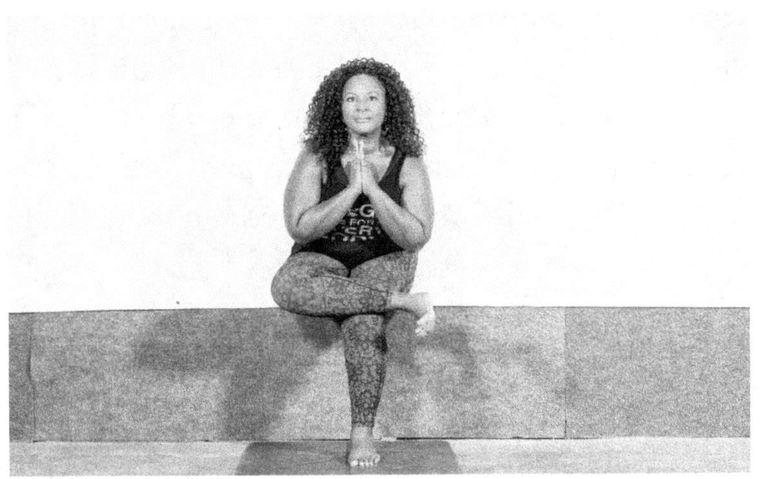

What is a wall squat?

A wall squat, often called a wall sit, is a bodyweight exercise that works the muscles in your core and lower body. To practice a wall squat, stand with your feet shoulder-width apart and your back flat against a wall. Lower yourself into a sitting position by bending your knees at 90 degrees. Keep your lower back firmly against the wall and hold the position for a specific amount of time.

If the activity is too tough, you can relieve stress in your low back by performing an exercise ball wall squat. In this variation, the identical steps are taken, but an exercise ball or stability ball is put between your lower back and the wall. If you want to increase the intensity of your workout, try a single-leg wall sit or a weighted dumbbell wall sit.

Benefits of Wall Squats

The wall squat provides several major advantages.

1. Wall squats increase core and lower-body strength. Wall squats are an excellent workout for strengthening your glutes, hamstrings, and quadriceps—particularly your inner thighs. Wall squats work your abdominal muscles as well as your legs, helping to increase core strength.

2. Wall squats increase physical endurance. Wall squats are an isometric exercise, which means the body stays in the same position throughout the session. Consistent repetition will enhance your muscular endurance, allowing you to hold the wall squat for longer periods of time.

3. Wall squats are a practical home exercise. Wall squats are among the most accessible and efficient leg exercises. They require no equipment and may be readily included into any training plan.

What's the difference between wall squats and standing squats?

Wall squats and standing squats have similar ranges of motion and engage the same muscle regions. However, there are a few significant variations between them.

Isometric vs. plyometric: Standing squats are plyometric exercises, whereas wall squats are isometric. This means that while doing wall squats, your body remains static, whereas standing squats keep your body moving.

Cardio level: While both exercises are good for strengthening your core and legs, standing squats will raise your heart rate more effectively and activate your cardiovascular system.

How to Perform Wall Squats with Correct Form

For wall squats, start with 2-3 sets of 30-60 seconds. Choose a time limit that will allow you to retain proper technique during each set.

1. Stand with your back to a solid wall and walk your feet forward. Your feet should be shoulder width apart.
2. Slide down the wall so that your thighs are parallel to the floor. Your knees should be over your ankles.
3. To ensure stability, evenly distribute your weight and grab the floor with your feet. Your upper body and head should rest against the wall.

Your chin should be tucked during the movement, as if you were cradling an egg under it.

4. Pretend your shoulders and hips while engaging your core. Your ribs should be lower and your pelvis somewhat tucked. Keep your arms at your sides or rest your hands on your legs. All repetitions should start from this position.

5. Maintain your alignment and full-body tension while holding the wall squat position for the specified amount of time.

6. Stand up, stretch, and do your chosen number of sets.

How to Exercise Safely and Avoid Injury

If you have a past or pre-existing health problem, speak with your doctor before starting an exercise program. Proper exercise technique is critical to the safety and efficacy of any exercise program, but you may need to adapt each exercise to achieve the best results based on your specific needs. Always choose a weight that permits you to maintain complete control of your body during the exercise. When undertaking any workout, pay great attention to your body and stop immediately if you feel pain or uncomfortable.

Incorporating adequate warm-ups, rest, and nutrition into your training regimen will help you make consistent progress and improve body strength. Your ability to recuperate properly from your workouts will ultimately determine your results. Rest for 24 to 48 hours before training the same muscle groups to allow for proper recovery.

Exercise 2: Wall Roll Down

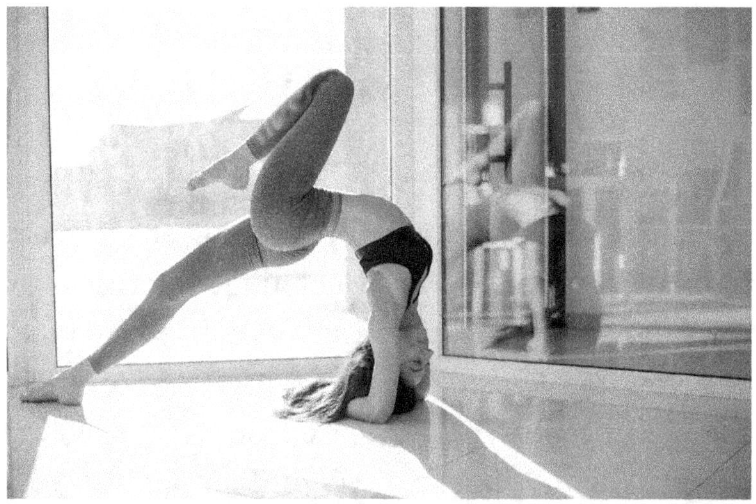

On personal experience and the advice of a teacher. Wall roll down is a basic standing mat workout. Practice using your abs to generate the articulated curve of the spine that is so common in Pilates. It stretches the back and hamstrings while working the abdominals and teaching proper posture. This is an effective approach to prepare for more difficult exercises such as the roll up, which requires the sequential activation of upper and lower abs to curl and uncurl the body. You might do it at home or as part of a warm up before a Pilates class.

Benefits

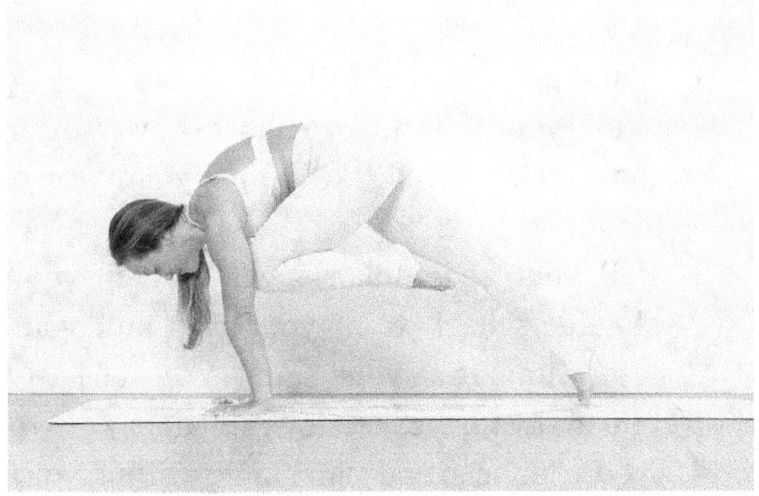

This exercise is ideal for Pilates beginners to develop engaging abdominals. In addition to working on the abs, you are also focused on relaxing the shoulders, which is where many individuals hold tension. You can use it to ease tension at any time of day. Poor posture is caused by hunched shoulders and strained neck muscles. Body awareness will help you improve your posture, take deeper breaths, and walk more comfortably. This will help to ease strain in your back, neck, hips, legs, and knees.

Step-by-step instructions.

1. Stand up against a wall.
2. Walk your feet 6 to 10 inches away from the wall while keeping your torso stationary.
3. Pull your abdominals inward. Keep your shoulders back from your ears and your arms straight at your sides. Your chest is big, and your ribs are low. Inhale.
4. Nod your head and start slowly rolling your spine down and away from the wall, vertebra by vertebra, while exhaling. As

you roll down, the abdominals remain raised, and you feel the spine extend. Your arms follow your body, remaining parallel to your ears. As the roll down develops, you can deepen the scoop of the abs even more. Work slowly to remove the spine away from the wall. Allow your head and neck to relax.

5. Roll as far down as you can without your hips leaving the wall. Inhale. Your abdominals are really tight. Feel the curvature evenly throughout your upper, middle, and lower torso. You might be getting a good hamstring stretch here.

6. Exhale and begin your return to the wall by rolling up with your lower abs. This is a powerful move. Consider engaging the lower abs to bring your pelvis upright. Continue up, putting each vertebra on the wall one by one.

7. As you get closer to upright, you'll notice a moment when you can keep your ribs down while your shoulders drop into position. It

feels as if your upper body is rolling up between your shoulders.

8. Bring your roll up to the starting position. Make sure your abs are engaged and your shoulders are lowered.

Common Mistakes

Avoid these mistakes to get the most out of this exercise while avoiding strain.

- **Going Too Fast.**
  This exercise should be done slowly, vertebra by vertebra, with control. Doing it at any speed will prevent you from feeling the connection.
- **Raised shoulders.**
  Make sure your shoulders are relaxed. Release the tension and become accustomed to this sensation, as it is vital for proper posture. You might want to check your Pilates posture.
- **Forcing the Stretch**

Do not push oneself to go lower than is comfortable. This isn't a toe touch. Roll as low as you can without causing the hips to leave the wall or strain.

Modifications and variations

There are modifications to this exercise that can make it easier to do as a novice while also deepening the experience.

Need a change?
Modify the wall roll down by only going as far as you feel comfortable. You may also bend your knees slightly.

Are you up for a challenge?
To alter this exercise, elevate your arms. Before beginning to roll down, extend your arms straight up over your head. While rolling down, maintain your arms parallel to your ears. As you roll up, your arms go alongside your ears while your shoulders remain relaxed. Finish with arms aloft, broad shoulders, and an open chest. The standing

roll down, done away from the wall, is another step forward.

Safety and precautions

Stop if you experience any pain throughout this activity. Roll as low as you can comfortably while maintaining contact with the wall. Because this exercise involves a small inversion, consult your doctor to see whether it is safe if you have glaucoma or high blood pressure. Stop if you become lightheaded or dizzy.

Exercise 3: Wall Push-Ups

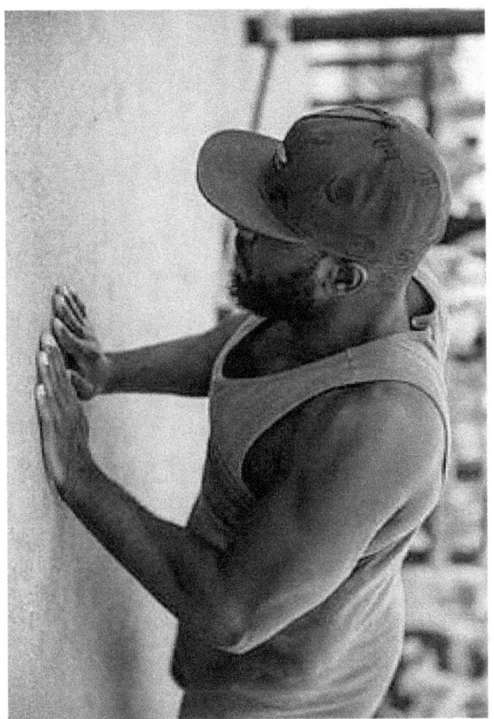

What are Wall Push-Ups?

Wall push-ups are a bodyweight workout that works the muscles in your arms, shoulders, and chests. To perform wall push-ups, stand in front of a wall with your feet shoulder-width apart and your hands against it; lean forward and bend your elbows, keeping your back and legs straight.

3 Advantages of Doing Wall Push-Ups

Regularly doing wall push-ups provides a few key advantages:

1. Wall push-ups are easier than regular push-ups. Standing during wall push-ups puts less strain on your shoulder joints and arms than regular push-ups, which need a plank position on the floor.
2. Wall push-ups increase upper-body strength. Wall push-ups, like regular push-ups, work muscles throughout the upper body, including the pectorals, anterior deltoids, and triceps.
3. Wall push-ups improve stability. Wall push-ups, when done correctly, work the midsection's stabilizer muscles, which include the abdominal and lower back muscles.

How to Perform Wall Push-Ups with Perfect Form

For wall push-ups, start with 2-3 sets of 15-20 repetitions. Choose the amount of sets and repetitions that will allow you to retain appropriate technique.

1. Start by standing arm's length from a wall.
2. Put your hands on the wall at shoulder height and slightly wider than your shoulders.
3. Take a step back with both feet. Your legs should be straight. Maintain your weight on the ball of your feet.
4. Rotate your shoulders outward to work your lats.MasterClass SEO Wall Push Up One
5. Squeeze your quadriceps and glutes while engaging your core. All repetitions should start from this position.MasterClass SEO Wall Push-Up TWO
6. Bend your elbows to lower your chest toward the wall. Your shoulder blades should retract while you move.
7. Lower your body so that your upper arms are level with your back.MasterClass SEO Wall Push Up THREE.
8. Pause for a second at the bottom of the exercise.

9. Squeeze your chest and straighten your elbows to start the upward movement while remaining in alignment.

10. Protract your shoulder blades as you push to the apex of the movement.

11. Complete the repetition by tightening your chest and triceps.

How to Exercise Safely and Avoid Injury

If you have a past or pre-existing health problem, speak with your doctor before starting an exercise program. Proper exercise technique is critical to the safety and efficacy of any exercise program, but you may need to adapt each exercise to achieve the best results based on your specific needs. Always choose a weight that permits you to maintain complete control of your body during the exercise. When undertaking any workout, pay great attention to your body and stop immediately if you feel pain or uncomfortable.

In order to see consistent growth and build body strength, include correct warm-ups, rest, and nutrition in your training routine. Your ability to recuperate properly from your workouts will ultimately determine your results. Rest for 24 to 48 hours before training the same muscle groups to allow for proper recovery.

Exercise 4: Wall Leg Lifts

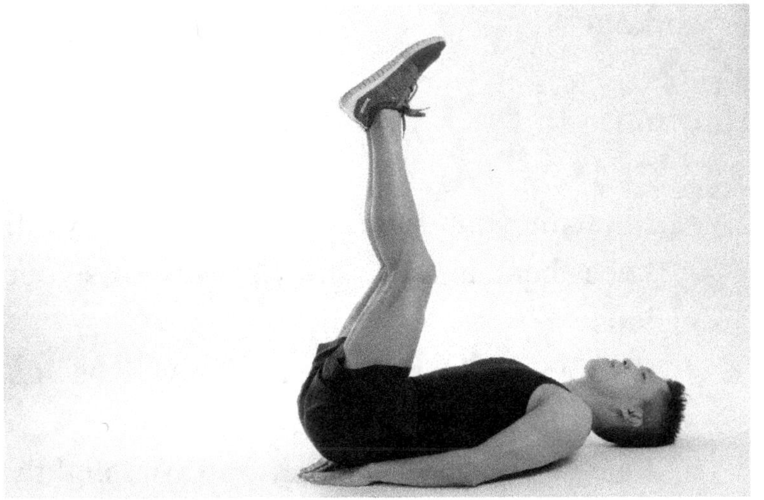

Legs-up-the-Wall Pose (Viparita Karani in Sanskrit) is a restorative yoga pose that can help reduce leg edema and varicose veins. However, there may be certain dangers for persons with specific conditions.

Legs-up-the-Wall Pose is an inversion yoga pose that elevates the hips and heart over the head. It is commonly used in Hatha, Yin, and Restorative yoga courses, but it can also be done on your own.

Legs-up-the-Wall Pose is accessible to a wide range of people due to its simplicity and versatility. It's ideal for those who are new to yoga or workout.

How to Do It

- Sit with your right side against the wall, knees bent, and feet drawn in towards your hips.
- Swing your legs up against the wall as you turn and lie flat on your back.
- Place your hips on the wall, or slightly away.
- Place your arms in a comfortable position.
- Stay in this position for 2–20 minutes.
- To exit the stance, carefully push yourself away from the wall.
- Relax on your back for a few moments.
- Draw your knees against your chest and roll to your right.

- Rest for a few moments before slowly returning to an upright position.

Variations

Once you've mastered Legs-up-the-Wall Pose, you may want to explore with new versions.

Butterfly

Bend your knees and bring the soles of your feet together in a Butterfly Pose (Wall Baddha Konasana). To increase the stretch, softly press your hands into your thighs. Alternatively, you might open your feet to the sides in a wide-legged position. You'll feel the stretch in your hips and inner thighs.

Wall Eye of the Needle Pose.

The Wall Eye of the Needle Pose provides a profound hip opening.

To do this:

- Begin with the Legs-up-the-Wall Pose, placing your legs on the wall and your back on the floor.
- Bend your right knee and position your outer ankle at the bottom of your left leg, just above the left knee.
- Slowly bend your left knee and press your foot on the wall.
- Lower your left foot so that your shin is parallel to the floor.
- You will experience a stretch in your right hip and thigh.
- Hold this position for 1-5 minutes.
- Repeat on the other side.

Other Things to Try

Consider the following suggestions to assist you find balance, a deeper stretch, or more lower back support while executing Legs-up-the-Wall Pose:

- Place a cushion, folded blanket, or bolster beneath your hips to promote flexibility.

- Bring your hips closer to the wall for a deeper stretch.
- To do pratyahara, bend your knees, position a pillow between them and the wall or beneath your head, and cover your eyes with a mask.
- Wrap a yoga strap over the base of your thighs to keep your legs in position.
- To practice breathing, lay a sandbag or weighted object on the bottoms of your feet and use diaphragmatic, equal, or resonant techniques.
- Use hand mudras, or hand poses, to help you stay calm and focused.

Benefits

There has been insufficient research into the specific benefits of the Legs-up-the-Wall Pose.

- The Legs-up-the-Wall Pose may provide psychological benefits such as lowering stress, anxiety, and tension.

- The authors of a 2020 study. According to Trusted Source's analysis of existing research, Legs-up-the-Wall Pose may also offer the following important benefits:
- Reduces leg swelling, weariness, and cramps, relieves sciatica pain, and prevents varicose veins.
- A 2024 review of researchAccording to a trusted source, Legs-up-the-Wall position may be a safe position for those with high blood pressure (hypertension) since it improves blood circulation and promotes lymphatic movement and drainage.

If you have hypertension, see a healthcare provider before doing inversion yoga positions. They may suggest other positions or cures.

Cautions

A 2023 study review.According to a trusted source, inversion yoga poses such as Legs-up-the-Wall can swiftly create pressure in the head and eyes. This could be a risk factor if you have an eye ailment like glaucoma. A tingling sensation in your legs and feet is a common side effect of elevating your legs high over your heart for an extended period of time. You might also feel like your legs and feet have gone asleep. If this happens, bend your knees into your chest before resuming the stance. You can also shake your legs to improve circulation.

Some people advise against inversions during the menstrual cycle, particularly on heavy-flow days. However, it is vital to highlight that scant evidence backs up these assertions. As a result, it is important to base your decision

CHAPTER 4

Intermediate Wall Pilates Exercises

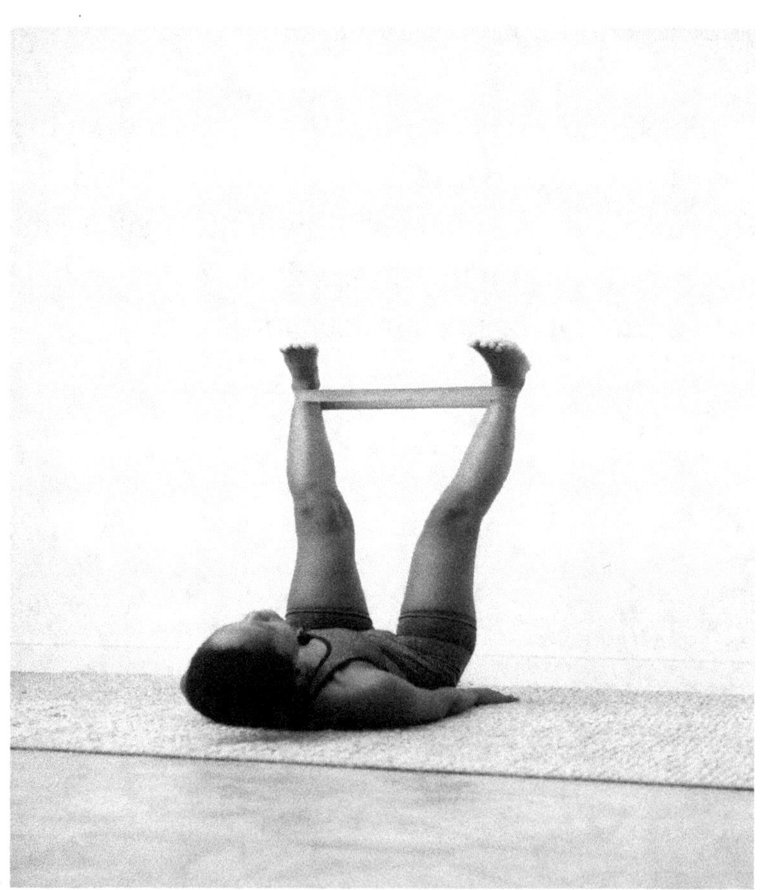

By now, you've constructed a strong basis with the fundamentals, and also you're geared up to elevate your practice to the next stage. These intermediate sports will mission your electricity, stability, and flexibility a chunk more, supporting your development at the same time as nevertheless using the wall as a aid device.

As always, do not forget to pay attention to your body. These moves are designed to boost your self assurance and manipulate, however you need to by no means push yourself to the factor of pain. Take it slow, recognize your breathing, and experience the advantages that include this conscious exercise.

What to Expect in Intermediate Exercises

In this chapter, we're going to construct on the foundation you've established with greater complex moves that will:

- **Increase electricity**: We'll specialize in activating deeper muscle tissue for your middle, legs, fingers, and back.
- These exercises will lightly challenge your flexibility, allowing you to deepen your stretches and improve your variety of movement.
- You'll expand higher stability as we contain movements that require balance and concentration.

Each exercise will continue to use the wall for support, but you'll also discover that your reliance on it is able to decrease as your stability and energy improve.

Exercise 1: Wall Angels

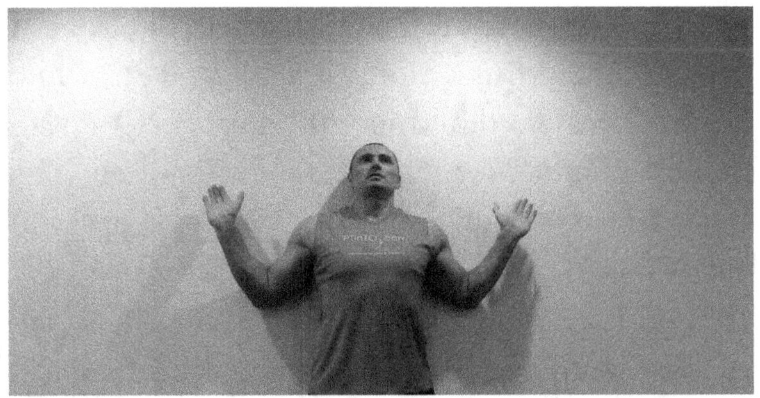

Many people today spend long periods of time sitting at a desk. In addition, sitting posture varies, frequently resulting in a depressed or contracted posture. There's also the dreaded "mobile cell phone posture," which requires a flexed posture whether you are sitting or standing.

When you sit for long periods of time, your lower back muscles keep your body in proper alignment. Eventually, these muscles weary, causing your body to droop and your head to tilt forward in reaction. Additionally, your trunk will flex and your pelvis will roll lower back. In reality, prolonged static postures, such as sitting at a computer or watching TV for an extended duration, might have an impact on your muscle electricity and period. The muscles in the back of your neck and trunk elongate and weaken, while the muscles in the front of your neck, chest, shoulders, and stomach tighten and shorten. The end result is a snowball effect, which keeps you in this posture even when you're no longer seated. The correct information? Performing targeted physical activities that strengthen your postural muscles can help combat this pattern.

Wall angels are an excellent choice. At this one exercise, you may strengthen your back muscles while also lengthening the muscle groups at the front of your neck, shoulders, and core.

What is a wall angel?

Wall angels are also known as a "V" to "W" stretch, which refers to the beginning and ending arm positions. They are normally performed with your back against a wall. The wall gives input to maintain your spine neutral and your arms in place.

This workout is beneficial if you sit most of the day or perform a lot of upper-body resistance training.

Exercises such as the bench press can cause muscles to shorten, but wall angels prevent this impact by stretching the chest muscles (pectoralis major and minor) and working the large back muscle (latissimus dorsi).

How to make wall angels.

1. Stand with your feet around 6-8 inches (15-20 cm) from the wall. Rest your buttocks, back, shoulders, and head against the wall.
2. Attempt to start with a neutral spine by drawing your belly button toward the spine. Draw your ribs in and down, allowing the rear of your ribcage to meet with the wall while keeping your lower back slightly away from it.

3. Tuck your chin slightly, aiming to make the back of your head touch the wall. If it's tough to place your head against the wall, consider placing a small pillow behind it.

4. Next, extend your arms straight up and place them on the wall overhead, aiming to have the back of your hands touch the wall in a "V" shape. If you are having trouble with any element of this alignment, move your feet further away from the wall and see if it resolves the problem.

5. Then, bend your elbows and glide your hands down the wall until they are just over your shoulders. Meanwhile, place your head, trunk, and buttocks against the wall.

6. Lower as much as possible while maintaining proper posture and avoiding pain. Hold for a count of 5 at the lowest point before returning to the "V" starting position with alignment intact.

7. Repeat 5-10 times, stopping when your muscles can no longer maintain the postural alignment without pain.

How to Modify:

If it is difficult to keep your spine against a wall without strain, you can perform this exercise while standing in a doorway rather than with your back against a wall.

To perform the modification, place your hands in the "V" posture on the edges of a doorway above your head. Step slowly through with one foot until you feel a stretch in your chest.

As with the traditional wall angel, draw your belly button in to bring your spine into neutral position, and slightly tuck your chin to keep your head as aligned with your torso as possible. Then, drop your hands down to the "W" position.

Return to your starting place and repeat. After 5-10 repetitions, take a step back and switch the lead foot.

This change will allow you to gradually improve your posture, making it easier to do angels against the wall in the future.

Benefits of Wall Angels

Wall angels activate postural muscles in your upper back, which assist maintain your shoulders pulled back. They also help to stretch and strengthen your chest, spine, and trunk muscles. Additionally, your core muscles must work to stabilize your trunk and keep you in a neutral position. As a result, they are an effective workout for counteracting the effects of a more contracted posture. This reduces stress in the shoulders, making it simpler to raise your arms overhead, and it keeps your head in line with your body, reducing stress in your neck muscles.

Common pitfalls when performing wall angels

During this exercise, your body may adjust in a variety of ways to allow you to reach overhead and drop your arms, resulting in incorrect form. The most popular is moving your buttocks away from the wall while slipping your arms overhead. This is usually caused by stiffness in the back, chest, and shoulder muscles. It could also be caused by tight hip flexors. To combat this, reduce your range of motion and avoid reaching as high until your flexibility improves.

Another problem is arching your back, which commonly happens during the lowering phase. This could be due to weak core stabilizing muscles or shoulder tightness. Again, limiting your range of motion and not dropping your arms as much will mitigate this.

Taking a forward-head position during the movement is another common compensatory strategy. This can happen when you raise or lower your arms, or during the entire movement. It is frequently caused by stiffness in the neck and chest muscles.

The fourth common mistake is failing to maintain hand and elbow contact with the wall. This is usually due to stiffness in the shoulders, chest, back, or trunk. This adjustment can also happen when you raise or drop your arms, or during the exercise.

Exercise 2: Wall Clamshells

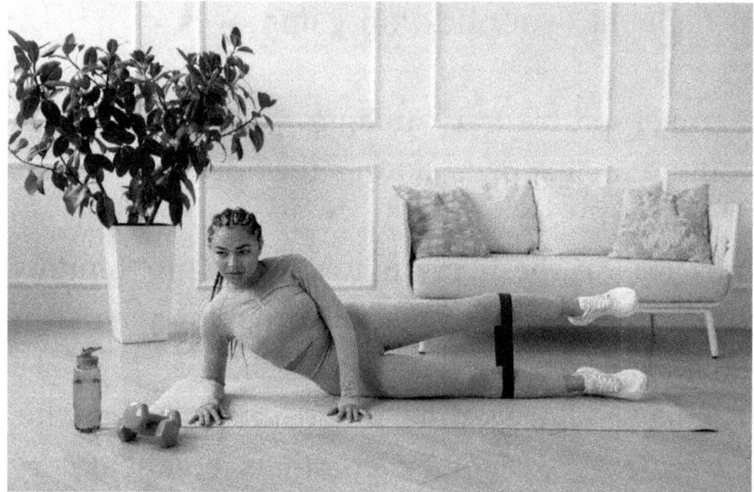

If you've been looking for an exercise that focuses your glutes while also improving your hip mobility, the clamshell exercise is the perfect solution. You've most likely seen the clamshell exercise in a Pilates class or during a strength-training session. While it appears simple after all, you're lying down — this one-of-a-kind action is popular among professionals across disciplines since it's a highly effective approach to develop hip strength, stability, and mobility. It's also versatile and customizable enough to fit easily into anyone's regimen, from novices to professional athletes. Ahead, we'll go over the benefits of the clamshell exercise, provide a step-by-step instruction for performing it correctly, and offer a few modifications to keep things interesting as you develop and build strength and mobility.

Clamshell Exercise Benefits

The clamshell exercise provides numerous advantages, including increased hip strength, stability, and overall lower-body function. It achieves this by focusing on the gluteus medius and minimus muscles, which are required for hip stability and abduction. According to studies from Stanford University's Sports Medicine Clinic, exercising these muscles can improve hip stability and lower the chance of future injury.

Additionally, clamshells can help correct muscle imbalances between the left and right sides of the body, which can lead to future problems. By targeting these muscles unilaterally, this exercise helps to minimize imbalances and create symmetry in the body. According to a 2015 Journal of Athletic Training research, workouts such as clamshells lower the risk of overuse injuries. Finally, one of the most significant advantages of this activity is its accessibility, which allows people of all fitness levels to participate. It may be readily customized by altering the range of motion or adding resistance with resistance bands or weights. Its simplicity makes it an excellent supplement to therapy strategies for patients healing from hip or knee problems.

How to Perform the Clamshell Exercise.

The clamshell appears to be, and indeed is, a simple movement. However, it relies on the mind-muscle link. You can just open and close your knees without working the glutes, missing out on the clamshell's powerful advantages. With that in mind, here's how to carry out the exercise properly and safely.

1. Come, lie on your side. Stack your hips on top of each other and bend your knees at a 45° angle.
2. Keeping your heels together, use your glutes to lift your top knee, opening your legs like a clamshell. Your knee should be raised toward the ceiling while also returning to the wall behind you. Keep your hips toward the wall in front of you.
3. Hold the position briefly at the peak, then gradually lower your leg back down while maintaining your glutes engaged. If you don't feel your glutes engaging during this movement, try warming up with one of these glute-activation exercises.
4. Repeat. Work your way up to 12 clamshells per side, for a total of three rounds.

Clamshell Exercise Variations:

Side Plank with Clamshell.

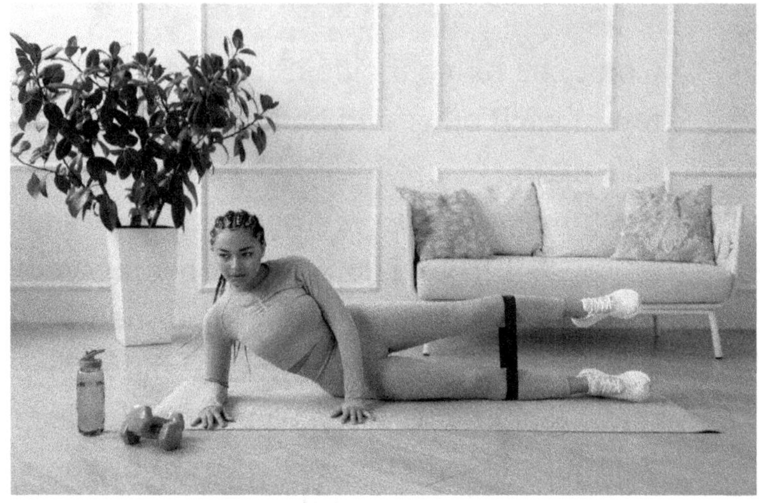

The addition of a bottom hip lift to the clamshell exercise, also known as a side bridge or side plank with a clamshell, increases the difficulty for the core and hip muscles.

1. Set up on your side, as you would with a standard clamshell.
2. Engage your obliques to raise your bottom hip off the ground. Create a straight line from your shoulders to your knees.

3. Lift your knee, using your glutes to assist the movement, as you would with a regular clamshell.
4. Hold the position briefly at the peak, then slowly lower your leg back down while keeping your hip elevated off the floor.
5. Repeat. Work your way up to 12 clamshells per side, for a total of three rounds.

Standing Clam Shell

To increase the difficulty, attempt a standing clamshell, often known as a squat walk. You may make this action more difficult by employing a hip band to provide resistance, requiring your glute muscles to work harder.

1. Bring your feet hip distance apart and squat down. To support the movement, engage your core and glutes.
2. Step your right foot further to the right while remaining in a squat.

3. Hold for a second, then move your left foot to the right to bring your feet back to hip width.
4. Repeat on the other side.
5. Perform 12 squat walks on each side, remaining in the squat position the entire time.
6. Continue with three rounds.

Copenhagen Plank

Copenhagen planks build strength in the abductors (outer thighs), hip flexors, and core, and its primary aim is the adductor muscles, making them an elevated version of the clamshell. It's a more complex maneuver, so start with a 10-second hold. Once you've mastered that, gradually increase the duration by five seconds.

1. Begin by lying on one side, with your forearm on the ground (left forearm if on the left side) and your shoulders stacked over your planted elbow.

2. Place your upper calf on a bench and your lower leg underneath it. This version requires both legs to be straight and parallel to one another.

3. Press against your leg on the bench and elevate your hips to align with your shoulders. As your hips raise, keep your shoulders stacked; you may find yourself rotating your upper shoulder in as you lift.

4. Lift your lower leg off the ground and bring it to meet the bench beneath. Hold this position.

5. Continue to press into your forearm to keep your core stable while lifting your body with your adductor.

6. Slowly lower yourself back to the floor beneath you.

Exercise 3: Wall Plank

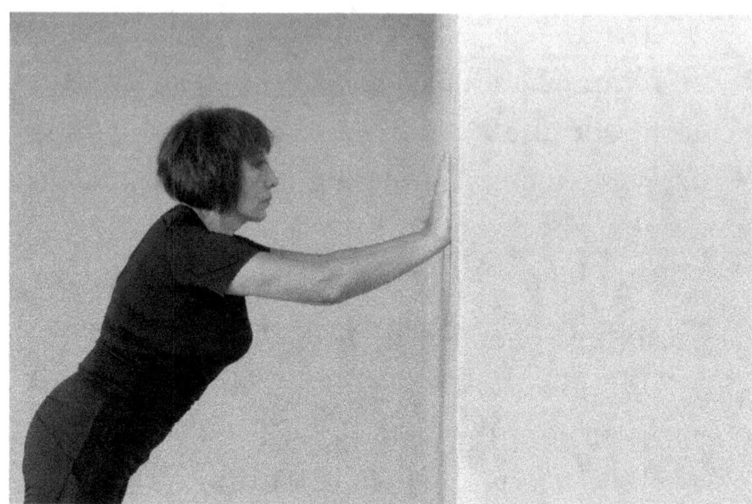

Are you weary of doing the same crunches and sit-ups but still want sculpted abs? Look no further! Wall planks are your secret weapon for shaping a rock-solid core, and they provide an intriguing option that produces excellent results. Wall planks have the ability to engage up to 80% more muscle fibers than standard exercises, making them a game changer in the realm of ab training. But be warned: this challenge is not for the faint of heart! It takes courage, determination, and persistence to master this powerful technique. If you're ready to sculpt those washboard abs and break free from the monotony, keep reading to learn about the remarkable benefits of wall planks and how they can transform your training regimen.

What is a Wall Plank?

A wall plank is a variation on the conventional plank exercise in which you support your body weight on a vertical surface, such as a wall. This difficult yet effective workout stimulates the same muscle groups as a typical plank, but with an added layer of challenge and engagement.

How are wall planks different from traditional planks? While both wall planks and standard planks are great exercises for training your abs, wall planks provide a more difficult challenge that involves more core stabilization and balance. Incorporating wall planks into your training program will offer diversity, intensity, and an edge to your core routines.

Wall Plank

Position: Your body forms a diagonal line with your feet on the ground and your hands or forearms against the wall.

Difficulty Level: The workout becomes more difficult as your body angle increases.

Core Engagement: Because maintaining balance and alignment is more challenging with wall planks, they need more core stabilization.

Variations: You can simply change wall planks by changing your body angle or integrating side wall planks to target oblique muscles.

Traditional Plank

Position: Your body is horizontal, with your toes on the ground and your forearms or hands supporting your upper body.

Difficulty Level: The difficulty of classic planks can be varied by moving your arms or legs.

Traditional planks work your core muscles, but they may not be as tough as wall planks in terms of balance and stabilization.

There are several varieties of classic planks, including side planks, reverse planks, and single-leg planks.

Which Muscles Do Wall Planks Use?

Wall planks primarily focus the core muscles, which are essential for spine stabilization, posture maintenance, and general physical performance. They also recruit supplementary muscle groups, which enhance the exercise's effectiveness.

Here's a breakdown of the primary and secondary muscles addressed by wall planks.
Major Muscles Targeted

1. Rectus Abdominis.
This muscle, located in the front of the abdomen, is also known as the "six-pack" muscle (2). During a wall plank, the rectus abdominis helps

to support your core and keep your body in a diagonal position. A strong rectus abdominis can help you perform better in exercises, lessen your risk of lower back pain, and support daily activities that require bending or twisting.

2. transverse abdominis

This deep abdominal muscle wraps around your torso like a corset and stabilizes the spine (2). In a wall plank, the transverse abdominis contracts to keep your body stable and in appropriate posture. Strengthening this muscle helps improve posture, core stability, and serve as a firm basis for subsequent exercises.

3. Obliques (Internal and External)

These muscles, positioned on the sides of your belly, aid in torso rotation and lateral flexion (2). While wall planks primarily target the core's frontal area, including side wall planks can effectively engage the obliques. Strong oblique muscles help to improve posture, rotational strength, and performance in sports and daily occupations that involve twisting motions.

Secondary Muscles Targeted

1) Deltoids

These shoulder muscles give stability and support during wall planks, particularly while your hands are against the wall. Strengthening the deltoids will help you maintain shoulder stability, avoid injuries, and perform better in upper body workouts like push-ups and overhead press.

2. Glutes.

During wall planks, the gluteus maximus, medius, and minimus muscles work together to stabilize your hips and keep them in perfect alignment. Strong glutes help balance, posture, and performance in lower-body workouts such as squats and lunges.

3) Quadriceps

These muscles, located at the front of your thighs, help keep your legs straight during wall planks.

Strengthening the quadriceps can help with overall leg strength, athletic performance, and daily activities like walking, running, and climbing stairs.

4. Erector Spinae.

These muscles go along the spine and help keep your back straight during wall planks. A strong erector spinae can improve posture, lower the risk of back pain, and provide critical support for other workouts requiring spinal stability.

How to Install a Wall Plank: Step-by-Step Instructions

1. Stand facing a solid wall, about 2-3 feet away.
2. Extend your arms and place your palms on the wall at shoulder height, shoulder-width apart. Ensure that your fingers are pointed upward.
3. Lean forward and move your weight to your hands, then walk your feet back until your body forms a diagonal line from your

head to your heels. Keep your feet hip width apart.

4. Draw your navel towards your spine to engage your core muscles. This will help you stay in perfect alignment and protect your lower back.

5. Keep your legs straight and your heels pressed into the ground for further support.

6. Hold your head in a neutral position with your eyes slightly downward, ensuring that your neck is in line with your spine.

7. Maintain even breathing throughout the workout, inhaling through your nose and expelling through your mouth.

8. Hold the wall plank posture for as long as possible while keeping perfect form, aiming for at least 30 seconds to begin. Gradually increase the duration as you gain strength.

If you find the normal wall plank too difficult, you can adjust it by standing closer to the wall or leaning your forearms against the wall rather than your hands. This minimizes your body's tilt and makes the exercise less intense.

How Long Should You Hold a Wall Plank?

The time you should hold a wall plank is determined by your current fitness level and ability to maintain good form. Beginners should strive to hold the wall plank for at least 30 seconds, focusing on proper alignment and muscle engagement. As your core strength and endurance develop, gradually extend your wall plank holds. Advanced exercisers can aim for 1-2 minutes or more, as long as appropriate technique is maintained during the workout.

Wall Plank Mistakes to Avoid and How to Correct Them

- **Sagging hips:** This typical mistake causes needless strain on the lower back. To correct it, activate your core muscles and concentrate on keeping a straight line from your head to your heels.

- **Piking hips:** Lifting your hips too high can make the workout less effective. Engage your core and glutes to maintain a diagonal line.
- Dropping your head causes tension on the neck and affects spinal alignment. Maintain a neutral head position, with your gaze slightly downward.
- **Holding breath:** Breathing incorrectly during a wall plank can produce dizziness and impair your ability to maintain the position. Throughout the workout, keep your breathing even and regulated.

Wall Plank Variations To Try

One-Arm Wall Plank
This version raises the difficulty by activating one arm at a time, necessitating greater core stabilization and balance.

<u>To do it:</u>

- Begin with the regular wall plank position.

- Slowly take one hand off the wall and lay it on your hip, or extend it straight to the side.
- Maintain appropriate form and alignment while holding the one-arm wall plank for 15-30 seconds.
- Return your hand to the wall and perform the exercise with your other arm.

Sidewall Plank

This variation focuses on the oblique muscles, offering a well-rounded core workout.

- Stand sideways against the wall, about 2-3 feet away.
- Place your forearm on the wall, keeping your elbow aligned with your shoulder.
- Extend your legs and stack your feet, resting on the wall with your body in a straight line.
- Hold the pose for at least 30 seconds with your core engaged.
- Switch sides and repeat the exercise.

Wall Plank with Leg Lift.

Adding leg lifts to your wall plank activates the glutes and lower back muscles, increasing the exercise and delivering a more complete workout.

To do it:

- Begin with the regular wall plank position.
- Slowly lift one leg off the ground while keeping it straight and in correct alignment.
- Hold the leg raise for 5 to 10 seconds before lowering it back down.
- Repeat with the opposite leg, switching legs for the appropriate number of times.

Wall Plank with Knee Tuck.

This variant targets the lower abs and hip flexors, providing an additional challenge to your core workout.

To do it:

- Begin in the regular wall plank position.
- Bend one knee and bring it to your chest without letting your hips drop or spin.
- Hold the knee tuck for around 2-3 seconds before lowering your foot to the ground.
- Repeat with the opposite leg, switching legs for the appropriate number of times.

Wall Plank with Shoulder Tap.

Adding shoulder taps to your wall plank promotes upper body activation and tests your balance.
<u>To do it:</u>

- Begin with the regular wall plank position.
- Slowly lift one hand from the wall and tap the opposing shoulder while maintaining your core engaged and solid.
- Return your hand to the wall and repeat the process with the opposite hand.
- Continue switching hands for the required number of repetitions, using proper form and alignment throughout the exercise.

- A lean, toned figure is not a pipe dream. Check out the BetterMe app and see how it can help you lose weight quickly.

Top Wall Plank Exercise Benefits:

Including wall planks in your workout has a lot of benefits, including:

Improved Core Strength
Wall planks work various core muscles, including the rectus abdominis, transverse abdominis, and obliques, leading to a stronger and more stable core.

Enhanced Balance and Stability
Wall planks increase balance, coordination, and overall stability by requiring you to maintain a diagonal position against the wall.

Better posture.
Strengthening the core muscles with wall planks improves posture by promoting good spinal

alignment and lowering the likelihood of slouching or hunching.

Increased flexibility
Wall planks stretch and lengthen a variety of muscles, including the shoulders, hamstrings, and calves, creating greater flexibility and mobility.

Reduced Lower Back Pain
A strong and stable core helps relieve stress on the lower back, potentially lessening discomfort and suffering caused by weak core muscles.

Full-Body Workout
Wall planks stimulate secondary muscle groups such as the deltoids, glutes, quadriceps, and erector spinae, making it an efficient total-body workout.

How Frequently Should You Do Wall Planks?

For best results, integrate wall planks into your workout regimen 2-3 times per week, with at least 48 hours between workouts for muscle recovery.

Including wall planks in a well-balanced fitness routine that targets multiple muscle groups can help prevent overtraining and muscular imbalances. Overdoing wall planks, or any workout, can have various harmful implications.

Muscle Fatigue

Performing wall planks too frequently without enough rest can lead to muscle fatigue, limiting your ability to maintain appropriate form and increasing your risk of injury.

Overuse Injuries.

Overworking the same muscle groups without enough rest time can result in overuse problems like strains, sprains, and tendonitis.

Decreased Performance

Overtraining can have a negative impact on your overall performance because muscles require time to rest and renew before being stronger.

Muscle Imbalances

Excessive focus on a single activity or muscle group can cause muscle imbalances, affecting posture, increasing the risk of injury, and impeding overall fitness progression.

To avoid these concerns, stick to a well-balanced training plan that targets different muscle groups while also allowing for proper rest and recovery. This will allow you to attain the best outcomes while reducing the danger of overtraining and injury.

Exercise 4: Wall Sit with Arm Raise

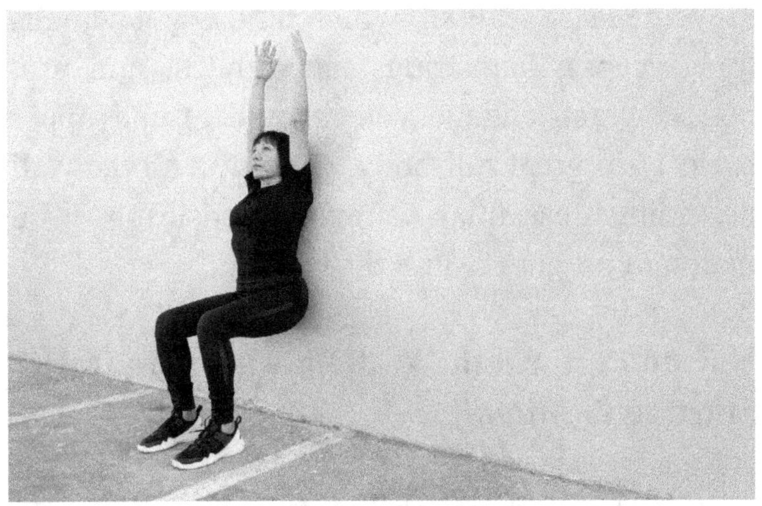

Wall Sit with Arm is a fantastic exercise that not only strengthens your lower body but also engages your upper body and improves overall endurance. As we age, maintaining strength in both the legs and arms is crucial for activities like walking, standing, and lifting. This exercise is gentle but effective, helping you build the endurance you need to stay active and independent.

Why Wall Sit with Arm Raise?

This exercise combines two important movements: a wall sit, which targets your thighs (quadriceps), hamstrings, and glutes, and arm raises, which engage your shoulders and upper back. It's a great full-body workout with the wall providing essential support, ensuring you maintain proper posture throughout.

How to Perform the Wall Sit with Arm Raise: Starting Position:

- Stand with your back against a sturdy wall, feet about hip-width apart, and about 18-24 inches away from the wall.
- Ensure your knees are in line with your toes, and your feet are facing forward.

Lower into a Wall Sit:
- Slowly slide your back down the wall, bending your knees until they are at about a 90-degree angle (or as low as feels comfortable).
- Keep your back pressed firmly against the wall and your core engaged. Your thighs

should be parallel to the ground, and your knees should not extend beyond your toes.

Raise Your Arms:
- As you hold the wall sit, inhale deeply, and as you exhale, raise your arms straight in front of you to shoulder height.
- Keep your arms straight but not locked at the elbows. You can also raise your arms overhead if your shoulders allow for the extra stretch.
- As you lift, focus on maintaining a neutral spine and tight core. Your upper body should stay relaxed, but engaged.

Hold and Breathe:
Hold the wall sit position while keeping your arms raised for 5-10 seconds (or longer if you're feeling strong!). Breathe slowly and steadily, allowing your muscles to work but staying relaxed in your movement.

Lower Your Arms and Rise:

- After holding the position, slowly lower your arms back to your sides as you inhale. Press through your heels and slide back up the wall to stand straight.
- Give your legs and arms a brief shake to release any tension.

Repetitions:

Aim for 8-10 repetitions, holding each wall sit and arm raise for 5-10 seconds. If you feel comfortable, gradually increase the hold time or the number of repetitions to build more strength and endurance.

<u>Tips for Success:</u>

1. **Posture is key:** Always keep your back pressed against the wall and your core engaged. This ensures that you're not putting unnecessary strain on your lower back or knees.

2. **Go at your own pace:** There's no need to rush! If holding the wall feels challenging at first, that's okay. Start with shorter holds

and gradually increase your endurance over time.

3. **Adjust for comfort:** If raising your arms overhead feels too strenuous on your shoulders, simply raise them to shoulder height. You can also keep your arms bent at the elbows if that feels more comfortable.

4. **Breathe steadily:** Inhale deeply as you prepare and exhale as you raise your arms. Controlled breathing helps you focus and ensures you're getting enough oxygen to fuel your muscles.

Benefits of the Wall Sit with Arm Raise:
1. The wall sit portion strengthens your quadriceps, hamstrings, and glutes, essential muscles for walking, standing, and overall mobility.
2. Raising your arms adds an extra challenge for your shoulders and upper back, improving endurance and coordination.
3. Keeping your back against the wall and your core engaged helps improve stability

and posture, which are key for preventing falls and maintaining balance.

4. This exercise is gentle on the joints, making it perfect for seniors looking to stay fit without putting too much stress on their knees or hips.

The Wall Sit with Arm Raise is a powerful yet gentle way to build strength, improve endurance, and increase mobility. Don't worry if it feels challenging at first — every hold you complete brings you one step closer to greater strength and stability. The key is consistency, so keep practicing and enjoy the rewards of your hard work! Remember, your body is capable of amazing things at any age. Stay committed, listen to your body, and keep moving forward.

CHAPTER 5

Advanced Wall Pilates Exercises

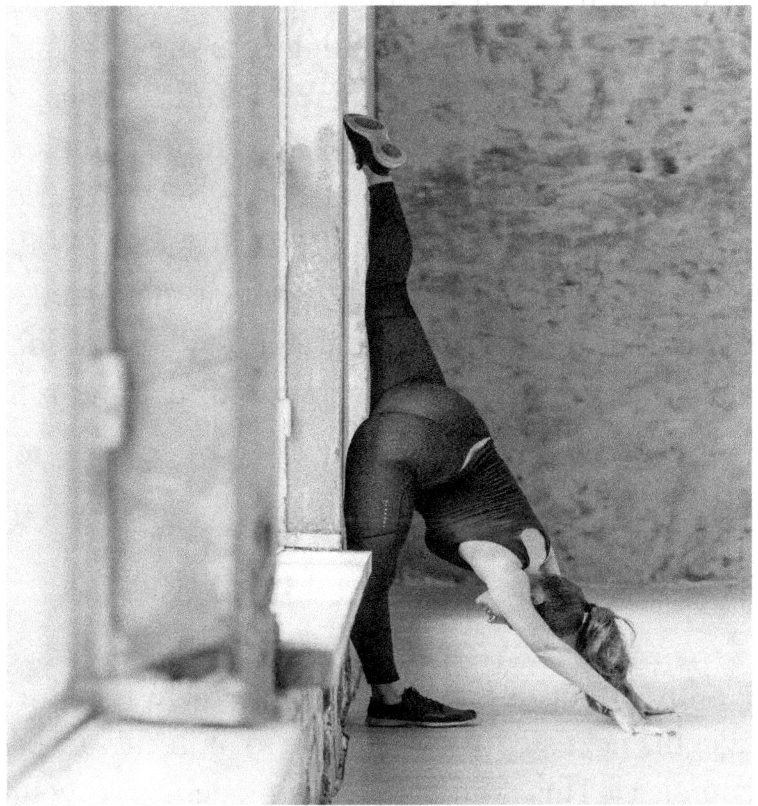

These advanced exercises are designed to challenge your strength, balance, and flexibility, helping you further enhance your mobility and overall well-being· As we move forward, remember that while these exercises are more demanding, the wall will continue to serve as your trusted support, which may allow you to push your limits safely· In this chapter, we'll focus on refining your form, building core strength, and increasing muscle endurance· You'll engage deeper muscle groups and work on more complex movements that will improve your posture, coordination, and stability· Advanced Wall Pilates is not about rushing through movements but rather about performing them with precision and control, allowing your body to reap the full benefits of the practice·

When to Move to Advanced Exercises

It's important to recognize when you're ready to take the next step and transition to more advanced exercises· This moment is about listening to your body, understanding your progress, and moving forward with confidence· Let's explore how to determine when you're ready to move from the basic and intermediate exercises to advanced ones, and what you should expect as you progress·

Signs You're Ready for Advanced Exercises:
1· Improved Strength and Endurance: If you've been consistently practicing the basics, you'll notice that your muscles, particularly in your core, legs, and back, feel stronger· You can hold positions like the Wall Sit or Wall Push-Up with more ease and for longer durations· This is a clear sign your body is ready for new challenges·
2· Increased Flexibility: Flexibility plays a crucial role in Pilates· If you've gained more flexibility in your spine, hips, and hamstrings through exercises like Wall Roll Down or Wall Squats, it's an indication you're prepared to explore movements that require deeper stretches and more control·
3· Better Balance and Coordination: Advanced exercises often incorporate more complex movements that require enhanced balance and coordination· If you feel more stable during exercises and can perform sequences with fluidity

and control, you're ready to introduce more challenging exercises·

4· Mastery of Form and Technique: When you can perform basic and intermediate exercises with proper form, alignment, and breathing, you're laying a solid foundation for more advanced movements· It's important to prioritize form over speed or intensity — moving into advanced exercises is all about maintaining that focus·

5· Physical and Mental Confidence: One of the most important indicators is how confident you feel during your workouts· If you find yourself finishing your sessions feeling strong, energized, and ready for more, that's a great sign that your body and mind are prepared for a new challenge·

What to Expect from Advanced Exercises:
- More Intensity: Advanced Wall Pilates exercises will push your strength and endurance further· You'll notice deeper engagement of your core, and your legs, arms, and back will be working harder·
- Complex Movements: You'll be combining movements and engaging

multiple muscle groups simultaneously·
These exercises will require focus and
control to maintain proper form and
balance throughout·
- Greater Flexibility and Range of Motion:
  Advanced exercises often incorporate a
  greater range of motion, asking your body
  to stretch further and bend deeper· Your
  flexibility will continue to improve as you
  progress through these movements·

A Few Reminders as You Progress:
- Pace Yourself: Just because you're ready
  for advanced exercises doesn't mean you
  have to master them all at once· Take your
  time and listen to your body· It's okay to
  start with fewer repetitions and gradually
  build up·
- Focus on Breathing: As exercises become
  more complex, it's even more important to
  maintain control over your breathing· Your
  breath will guide the movement and help
  you sustain energy throughout the
  workout·

- Don't Forget the Basics: Always return to foundational exercises when needed· The basics are your building blocks, and revisiting them will help keep your form sharp and ensure you're performing advanced movements safely and effectively·

- Modify When Necessary: If any of the advanced exercises feel too challenging, don't hesitate to modify them· It's important to honor your body's needs and work within your comfort zone to avoid injury·

Moving into advanced exercises is an exciting milestone in your Wall Pilates journey· It reflects the progress you've made in building strength, flexibility, and confidence· These exercises will challenge you in new ways, pushing you to grow stronger and more in tune with your body· Remember, the key to Pilates at any level is mindfulness and precision· Embrace this new chapter, stay patient with yourself, and celebrate your hard work· Your dedication is paying off, and you are proving that no matter your age, you can continue to grow, improve, and thrive!

Exercise 1: Wall Side Leg Raise

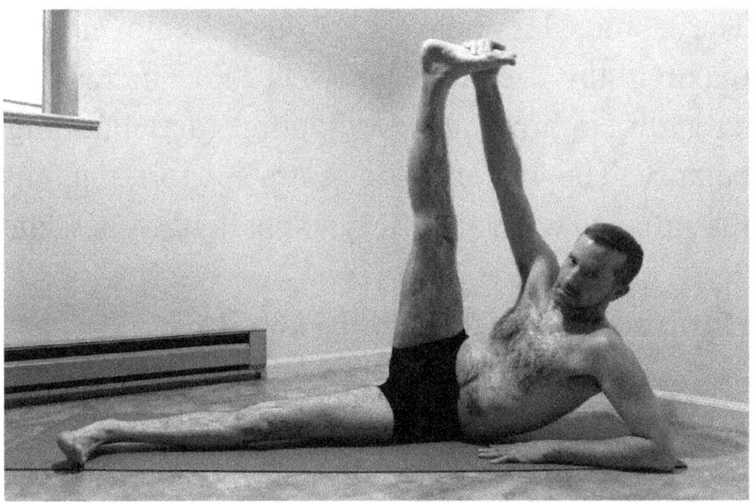

Wall Side Leg Raise is an effective and targeted exercise to strengthen your hip muscles, improve balance, and enhance overall lower body stability· As we age, maintaining strong hips is essential for mobility, balance, and preventing falls· This gentle yet powerful movement helps keep your legs and hips strong, flexible, and mobile, making everyday activities like walking and climbing stairs easier and safer·

Why Wall Side Leg Raise?

The Wall Side Leg Raise specifically targets your hip abductors, muscles that are vital for stabilizing your pelvis and improving balance· These muscles help with lateral movement, making this exercise perfect for increasing strength, improving coordination, and building balance· The wall provides extra support, making it a safe and controlled way to challenge yourself·

How to Perform Wall Side Leg Raise:

1· **Starting Position:** Stand sideways next to a wall, about an arm's length away, with your feet hip-width apart· Place your hand on the wall for support· If you'd like, place your other hand on your hip to help maintain balance· Engage your core and keep your posture tall, shoulders back, and chest open·

2· **Lift the Leg:** Inhale to prepare· As you exhale, slowly raise the leg that's farthest from the wall out to the side· Keep your leg straight but soft at the knee· Lift your leg to a comfortable height no need to lift too high· Focus on keeping your movement controlled and steady·

3· Hold and Balance: Hold the leg raise for 1-2 seconds, feeling the muscles in your outer hip engage· Keep your toes pointed forward and avoid tilting your body to the side·

4· Lower the Leg: Inhale as you gently lower your leg back to the starting position, maintaining control throughout the movement·

Repeat the lift and lower, maintaining your balance and using the wall as needed·

5· Switch Sides: After completing the desired repetitions, turn around and repeat the exercise on the other side to balance out your workout·

Repetitions:

Perform 8-12 repetitions on each side· As you grow stronger, you can add more repetitions or hold the leg raise for a longer duration·

Tips for Success:

- **Engage Your Core:** Keep your abdominal muscles engaged throughout the exercise to help stabilize your body and protect your lower back·

- **Maintain Proper Alignment:** Avoid leaning into the wall or tilting your torso to one side· The goal is to keep your body upright and let the work come from your hip and leg muscles·

- **Move Slowly and With Control:** It's not about how high you can lift your leg, but about performing the movement with control and precision· Slow, steady movements are key to activating the right muscles·

- **Breathe:** Inhale as you lower your leg, exhale as you lift· Controlled breathing helps you stay focused and ensures that you're engaging your muscles properly·

Benefits of the Wall Side Leg Raise:

- Strengthens Hip Muscles: This exercise directly targets your hip abductors, helping to improve the strength and flexibility of the hips and legs·

- Improves Balance: By performing this single-leg exercise, you challenge your balance, which is key to preventing falls and staying independent as you age·
- Enhances Lower Body Stability: Stronger hips lead to better pelvic stability, making it easier to maintain good posture and balance in everyday activities·
- Gentle on the Joints: This low-impact exercise is ideal for seniors, as it's easy on the joints but still effective at building strength and endurance·

The Wall Side Leg Raise is a simple yet powerful exercise to keep your hips strong, flexible, and stable· Don't worry if your leg lift feels small at first, every repetition you complete strengthens those important muscles and helps improve your balance· With regular practice, you'll notice greater stability in your daily movements and increased confidence in your ability to stay active and mobile· Remember, consistency is key· Keep practicing, focus on maintaining proper form, and enjoy the benefits of a stronger, more stable lower body·

Exercise 2: Wall Single Leg Squat

This exercise is a great way to challenge your balance, strengthen your legs, and improve the stability of your lower body· As we age, maintaining strength in our legs is crucial for everyday activities like walking, climbing stairs, and standing up from a chair· The Wall Single Leg Squat helps target the muscles that keep you mobile and independent, while the wall provides the support you need to feel confident in every movement·

Why Wall Single Leg Squat?
The Wall Single Leg Squat targets your quadriceps, hamstrings, and glutes — the major muscle groups in your legs· It also works your core and hip stabilizers, which are important for balance and posture· This exercise allows you to

safely practice single-leg movements, a key skill for improving overall stability and reducing the risk of falls· Plus, the wall offers extra support, making it ideal for seniors who want to strengthen their lower body without putting too much pressure on their joints·

How to Perform Wall Single Leg Squat:
1· **Starting Position:** Stand with your back against a wall and your feet hip-width apart·
Step your feet out about 12-18 inches from the wall, so your body forms a slight angle with the wall· Lift your right leg slightly off the floor, keeping your weight balanced on your left leg· You can keep your hands at your sides or extend them in front of you for extra balance·
2· **Squat Down:** Inhale to prepare· As you exhale, slowly bend your left knee and lower your body into a squat position, allowing your back to slide down the wall· Go as low as feels comfortable for you, aiming to form a 45-degree angle or slightly lower at the knee· Keep your lifted leg straight, and try not to let your supporting knee extend past your toes·

3· **Hold and Engage:** Hold the squat position for a brief moment, focusing on engaging your core and leg muscles· The goal is to maintain balance and control throughout the movement.

4· **Stand Back Up**: Inhale as you press through your left heel and slowly straighten your leg to return to a standing position· Make sure to keep your core engaged and avoid locking your knee as you come back up·

5· **Switch Sides:** Once you've completed the repetitions on your left leg, switch to your right leg and repeat the movement, ensuring balance between both sides·

Repetitions:

Perform 5-8 repetitions on each leg· As you become stronger and more comfortable with the exercise, aim to increase the number of repetitions or hold the squat for a longer duration·

Tips for Success:

- Engage Your Core: Your core muscles are key to maintaining balance in this exercise·

Keep them activated throughout the movement to help stabilize your body·

- Keep Your Knees Aligned: Make sure your knee stays in line with your toes when you squat· Avoid letting your knee cave inward or extend too far over your toes·
- Use the Wall for Support: Don't be afraid to use the wall to help you control your movements· It provides the extra stability you need to focus on building strength in your legs without worrying about falling·
- Modify as Needed: If the single-leg squat feels too challenging at first, start by lowering yourself only part of the way· As your strength improves, you can deepen the squat·

Benefits of the Wall Single Leg Squat:
- **Strengthens Leg Muscles:** This exercise focuses on the quadriceps, hamstrings, and glutes, helping to build strength in the legs for improved mobility·
- **Improves Balance and Stability:** By practicing single-leg movements, you

challenge your balance and coordination, which is important for preventing falls and maintaining independence·

- **Builds Functional Strength:** Strengthening your legs and improving your balance through the Wall Single Leg Squat can make everyday tasks easier, from standing up from a chair to climbing stairs·

- **Gentle on Joints:** The wall provides support, reducing the pressure on your knees and hips, making this a safe and effective exercise for seniors·

The Wall Single Leg Squat is a fantastic exercise for building lower body strength, enhancing balance, and improving overall stability· By practicing this movement regularly, you'll gain more confidence in your legs and core, helping you stay active and mobile in your daily life· Take your time with this exercise and focus on slow, controlled movements· It's okay if your squat isn't deep at first every time you perform this exercise, you're building strength and improving your form· Remember to stay mindful of your body, keep your movements smooth, and most importantly, have fun with it·

Exercise 3: Wall Pike

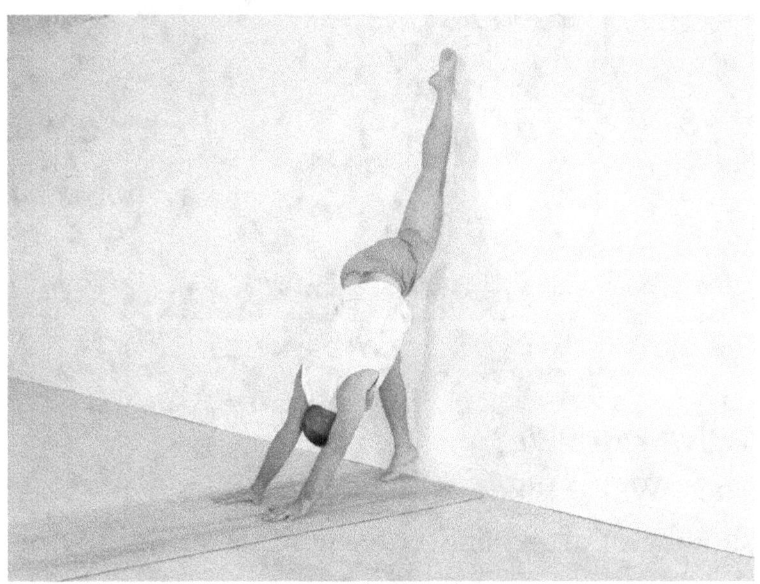

Wall Pike is a fantastic exercise that will challenge your flexibility, engage your core, and help you build strength in your upper body· This movement is a combination of a stretch and a strength exercise, making it an excellent addition to your Wall Pilates routine· The Wall Pike will improve your shoulder mobility, strengthen your arms, and stretch your hamstrings, all while giving your core a fantastic workout·

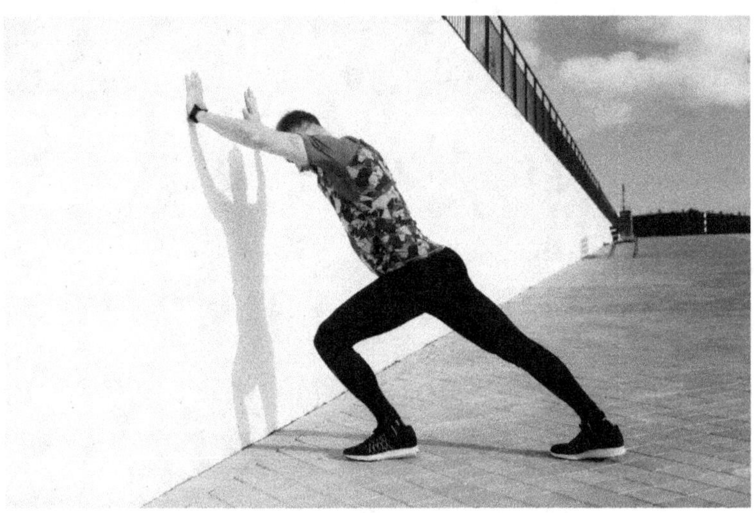

Why Wall Pike?

The Wall Pike works to strengthen your shoulders, arms, and core, while also improving flexibility in your hamstrings and lower back· This exercise helps enhance your overall body awareness and control, while the wall provides support to keep the movement safe and accessible for seniors· It's a great way to stretch and tone your muscles while improving balance and coordination·

How to Perform Wall Pike:

1· Starting Position: Stand facing the wall, about an arm's length away· Place your hands on the wall at shoulder height, palms flat, and fingers pointing upwards· Walk your feet backward, keeping them hip-width apart, until your body forms an "L" shape, with your torso parallel to the floor· Keep your back flat and your core engaged· Your legs should be straight but soft at the knees, and your arms should be fully extended in front of you, creating a strong line from your hands to your hips·

2· Pike Position: Inhale deeply, then as you exhale, begin to slowly press your hips upward toward the ceiling· As you lift your hips, allow your head to drop gently between your arms, keeping your neck in line with your spine· Your body should form an inverted "V" shape, with your tailbone pointing up and your heels pressing gently toward the floor· Focus on maintaining length in your spine and keeping your shoulders engaged·

3· Hold and Stretch: Hold the Pike position for a few breaths, feeling the stretch in your hamstrings, shoulders, and lower back· Focus on deep, steady breathing to help release any tension in your muscles· Keep your core engaged throughout the movement to support your lower back and maintain balance·

4· Return to Starting Position: To come out of the Pike, inhale and slowly lower your hips back down to the starting "L" shape position, walking your feet forward slightly if needed·

Keep your core tight and move with control to avoid any strain on your shoulders or back·

Repetitions:

Hold the Pike position for 10-20 seconds, then return to the starting position· Perform 3-5 repetitions, focusing on maintaining control and balance throughout the movement·

<u>Tips for Success:</u>

- **Engage Your Core:** This exercise requires a lot of core engagement to maintain stability and protect your lower back· Keep your abdominal muscles pulled in throughout the movement·

- **Move Slowly and With Control:** As you move into and out of the Pike position, go slowly and focus on maintaining proper form· This ensures you're getting the most benefit from the exercise while reducing the risk of injury·

- **Keep a Neutral Spine:** Make sure to keep your back flat and avoid arching or rounding your spine· This helps you stay aligned and prevents any unnecessary strain on your back·

- **Modify if Needed:** If the full Pike feels too intense, you can modify the exercise by keeping your knees slightly bent or performing the movement at a higher angle· The goal is to find a position that feels comfortable and allows you to perform the exercise with good form·

Benefits of the Wall Pike:

- **Strengthens Upper Body and Core:** This exercise engages your arms, shoulders, and core, helping to build strength and stability in these key areas·
- **Improves Flexibility:** The Wall Pike provides an excellent stretch for your hamstrings, lower back, and shoulders, helping to improve flexibility and range of motion·
- **Enhances Balance and Coordination:** As you move through the Pike position, you'll need to maintain control and balance, which helps improve your coordination and body awareness·
- **Gentle on the Joints:** The Wall Pike is a low-impact exercise, making it a great option for seniors who want to build strength and flexibility without putting excessive strain on their joints·

The Wall Pike is a wonderful exercise that combines strength, flexibility, and balance in one fluid movement· As you practice this exercise, you'll notice improved mobility in your shoulders and hamstrings, stronger arms, and a more engaged core· Don't rush the movement — take your time, focus on your breath, and enjoy the stretch and strength that comes with each repetition· With consistent practice, the Wall Pike will help you build a strong and flexible body, making everyday activities easier and keeping you feeling energized· Remember, you're doing amazing, and every time you perform this exercise, you're investing in your long-term strength and well-being·

Exercise 4: Wall Arm Circles

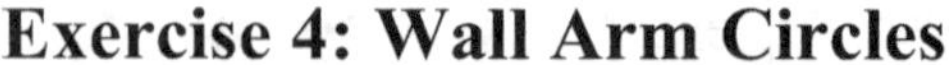

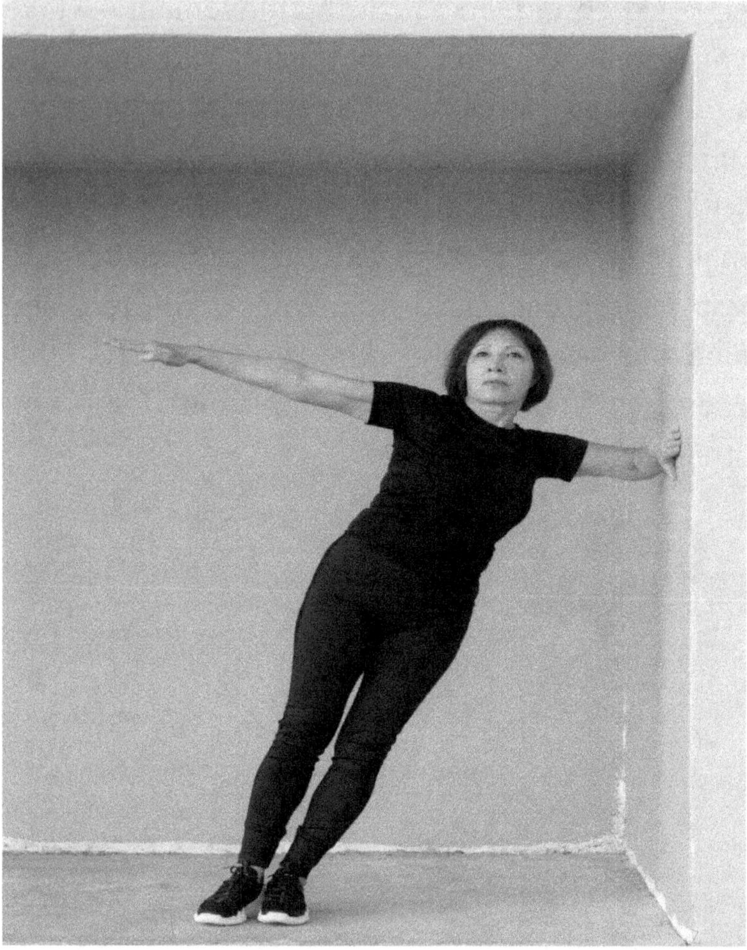

This simple yet effective movement is designed to strengthen your shoulders, improve your range of motion, and enhance flexibility in your upper body· As we age, maintaining mobility in our shoulders and arms is essential for everyday activities like reaching, lifting, and even maintaining good posture· The Wall Arm Circles exercise offers a low-impact way to improve shoulder joint mobility while gently strengthening the surrounding muscles·

Why Wall Arm Circles?

The Wall Arm Circles specifically target the shoulder muscles and rotator cuff, improving shoulder flexibility and strength· This exercise also engages your upper back and arms, helping to relieve stiffness and improve circulation in your upper body· It's a great way to warm up your shoulders and prevent injury, especially if you experience tightness or discomfort in this area· The support of the wall ensures that you can perform the exercise with stability, making it safe and accessible for seniors·

How to Perform Wall Arm Circles:

1· **Starting Position:** Stand facing the wall, about an arm's length away· Place your palms flat against the wall at shoulder height, keeping your arms straight but not locked· Keep your feet hip-width apart and maintain a soft bend in your knees to ensure good posture· Engage your core to stabilize your upper body·

2· Small Circles: Inhale to prepare· As you exhale, begin making small circular motions with your hands on the wall· Move your hands in a forward circular motion, starting with slow, controlled circles· Focus on keeping your arms straight and shoulders down, away from your ears· Your hands should stay connected to the wall as you make the circles·

3· Reverse the Circles: After completing a set of forward circles, switch directions and start making circles in the reverse direction, moving backward with the same control and pace· Remember to keep your core engaged and avoid arching your back as you move· The motion should come from your shoulder joints, not from your torso·

4· Increase the Circle Size: As your shoulders warm up and become more comfortable with the movement, you can gradually increase the size of the circles· Start with smaller circles, then make them slightly larger if your range of motion allows·

Repetitions:

Perform 10-15 circles in each direction (forward and reverse)· Take your time and ensure smooth, controlled movements· If you feel tension or tightness in your shoulders, you can stick with smaller circles until you feel more comfortable·

Tips for Success:

- **Engage Your Core:** Keep your abdominal muscles activated to maintain good posture and prevent any strain on your lower back·
- **Keep Shoulders Down:** Avoid raising your shoulders toward your ears· Focus on keeping your shoulders relaxed and down throughout the exercise to promote proper alignment·
- **Move With Control:** Slow, controlled movements are key· Don't rush the circles lct your shoulder joints guide the movement, and avoid jerky motions·

- **Modify as Needed:** If you experience any discomfort or reduced mobility, you can make the circles smaller or limit the range of motion to what feels comfortable· Over time, your flexibility will improve·

Benefits of the Wall Arm Circles:

- **Improves Shoulder Flexibility:** This exercise helps increase the range of motion in your shoulders, making daily tasks like reaching and lifting easier·
- **Strengthens Upper Body Muscles:** Wall Arm Circles target the shoulder muscles and rotator cuff, which are essential for upper body strength and stability·
- **Enhances Circulation:** The movement promotes blood flow to your shoulders and arms, which helps relieve tension and stiffness·
- **Prevents Shoulder Injuries:** By gently mobilizing your shoulders, you reduce the risk of injury and improve joint health, which is especially important as we age·

- **Safe and Accessible:** The support of the wall makes this exercise ideal for seniors, as it allows you to focus on proper form without worrying about balance or stability·

The Wall Arm Circles are a simple yet highly effective way to improve flexibility, relieve shoulder tension, and maintain upper body strength· Whether you're warming up for more exercises or simply want to improve your shoulder health, this exercise is perfect for keeping your shoulders mobile and strong· Remember, consistency is key· The more you practice, the more you'll feel your range of motion increase, and you'll find it easier to perform everyday tasks with less effort and strain· Take your time, focus on controlled movements, and celebrate every bit of progress· You're doing fantastic! Keep up the great work, and let's keep those shoulders moving freely!

CHAPTER 6

Customizing Your Workout

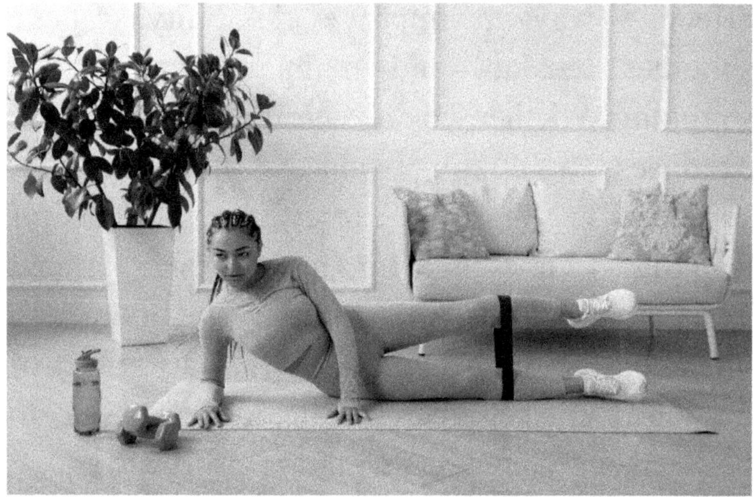

At this stage, you should have mastered the fundamentals of Wall Pilates, and now it's time to tailor your routine to suit your unique needs and fitness goals. As a Wall Pilates coach, I'm here to remind you that everyone's body is different, and that's something to celebrate! The beauty of Wall Pilates is that it's adaptable, allowing you to make adjustments that ensure you're getting the most out of every exercise, while staying safe and comfortable. Our bodies change over time, and what works best for someone else might not be the perfect fit for you. By customizing your workout, you can focus on areas where you want to build strength, improve flexibility, or enhance balance. Maybe your knees feel a bit stiff, or perhaps you want to spend extra time on core stability, customizing your workout lets you focus on what matters most for you.

Creating a Personalized Routine

As your Wall Pilates coach, I'm here to remind you that one size does not fit all, especially when it comes to your fitness routine· Creating a personalized workout plan is the key to achieving your goals, staying motivated, and making sure you're moving in ways that feel right for your body· Whether you're looking to build strength, improve flexibility, or boost balance, your personalized Wall Pilates routine should reflect your current abilities and individual goals·

Step 1: Identify Your Goals

The first step in personalizing your routine is to focus on what you want to achieve· Ask yourself:

- Do you want to strengthen a particular area? Maybe you want to focus on your core, or perhaps your legs need more attention·
- Are you looking to improve flexibility? If you feel stiffness in your hips or lower back, it might be time to incorporate more stretching exercises·
- Do you want to improve balance or coordination? Balance is key to maintaining independence and preventing falls, so exercises that challenge stability can be an excellent focus·

Once you have a clear picture of your goals, you can begin building your routine with exercises that target those specific areas·

Step 2: Choose Your Exercises

Now that you've identified your goals, it's time to choose the exercises that will help you reach them· For instance:

- If strength is your goal, exercises like Wall Push-Ups, Wall Squats, and Wall Leg Lifts are excellent choices·
- If flexibility is what you're after, focus on Wall Roll Downs and Wall Pike to stretch and lengthen your muscles·
- For balance, incorporate exercises like Standing Leg Circles or Wall Planks that challenge your stability·

Make sure to include a variety of movements to work different muscle groups, and always start with a warm-up to get your body moving·

Step 3: Adjust Repetitions and Sets

Your workout should be challenging but achievable· As a beginner, you may start with just 5 to 8 repetitions of each exercise, gradually increasing the number as you get stronger and more comfortable· Typically, completing 2 to 3 sets of each exercise is a good starting point, but you can adjust based on your energy level and how you feel·

Modifying Exercises for Comfort and Safety

Wall Pilates is all about control and precision, but it's also about moving in a way that feels comfortable and safe· Modifying exercises ensures that you are working within your limits while still reaping the benefits· Let's explore how to modify some key exercises to suit your body:

1· Adjusting Range of Motion

If you feel tightness in your joints or muscles, it's okay to reduce the range of motion· For example:

During a Wall Squat, don't feel the need to squat too deeply if your knees feel uncomfortable· A small, controlled bend will still engage your muscles· For a Wall Push-Up, you can bring your hands closer to the wall, reducing the distance you have to push, to ease the pressure on your shoulders·

2· Use Props for Support

You can always make adjustments by using props to support your movements:

Place a pillow or rolled-up towel behind your back during exercises like Wall Roll Downs to provide extra support if you experience any discomfort· If you find balance challenging during standing exercises, use a chair for stability until you feel more confident· This modification keeps you safe while still allowing you to challenge your balance gradually·

3· Listen to Your Body

One of the most important aspects of Pilates, especially for seniors, is learning to listen to your body· If an exercise causes discomfort or pain, stop and modify· Pain is never a goal in Pilates—strengthening and stretching safely is· If you feel tired or strained, take a break, slow down, or reduce the intensity· Remember, you're in control·

Staying Safe While Progressing

Progress takes time, and it's essential to go at your own pace· Over time, your strength, flexibility, and balance will improve, allowing you to take on more challenging exercises or increase your repetitions· But always prioritize safety:

- Warm up before every session to get your body moving and prevent injury·
- Hydrate to keep your body functioning at its best·
- Breathe steadily throughout each exercise to stay relaxed and focused·
- If you're ever unsure, ask a professional or use this book's guidance to modify an exercise for your comfort·

Remember, it's not about how fast you move or how deeply you stretch—it's about doing what's right for your body each day· Customization is key to building a sustainable fitness routine that serves you now and into the future· With every session, you're investing in your health and well-being, so feel proud of each step you take· You're moving at the right pace for you, and that's something to celebrate·

Combining Exercises for Full-Body Workouts

When you combine exercises, you can maximize the benefits while keeping your workouts engaging and fun·

Why Combine Exercises?
Combining exercises is a fantastic way to:

- **Increase Efficiency:** By targeting multiple muscle groups in a single session, you can achieve more in less time· This is especially beneficial for seniors who want to maintain their fitness without dedicating excessive hours to exercise·
- **Enhance Coordination:** Working different muscle groups together improves your coordination and balance, which are essential for daily activities and maintaining independence·

- **Boost Motivation:** A varied routine keeps things interesting! Mixing exercises helps prevent boredom and can motivate you to stick with your practice·

Creating Your Full-Body Workout

1· Warm-Up (5-10 minutes): Begin with gentle movements like Wall Roll Downs to warm up your spine and shoulders· Follow up with Wall Arm Circles to activate your shoulder joints and improve mobility·

2· Choose Your Exercises: Select a combination of exercises that target different muscle groups· Here's a sample workout you can try:

- Wall Squats (Legs and Glutes): Stand with your back against the wall and slide down into a squat· Hold for a few seconds, then rise back up· Repeat 10-15 times·
- Wall Push-Ups (Chest and Arms): Place your hands on the wall at shoulder height and perform push-ups· Aim for 8-12

repetitions, focusing on controlled movements·

- Wall Leg Lifts (Core and Legs): Stand facing the wall and lift one leg to the side, keeping it straight· Alternate legs for a total of 10-12 lifts on each side·
- Wall Plank (Core Stability): Place your forearms on the wall and walk your feet back to form a straight line from head to heels· Hold this position for 15-30 seconds·
- Standing Roll Down (Spinal Flexibility): Stand tall, take a deep breath in, and as you exhale, roll down vertebra by vertebra, reaching toward your toes· Roll back up slowly· Repeat 3-5 times·

3· Cool Down (5-10 minutes):
Finish your session with gentle stretches like the Wall Chest Stretch and Wall Calf Stretch to promote flexibility and relaxation·

Tips for Staying Motivated

Staying motivated is crucial to maintaining a consistent Wall Pilates practice, especially as we age· Here are some effective strategies to help you stay on track and keep your enthusiasm high:

1· Set Realistic Goals: Start with small, achievable goals that can lead to significant progress over time· Whether it's increasing your flexibility, completing more repetitions, or simply committing to three sessions a week, setting goals gives you something to work towards·

2· Track Your Progress: Keep a journal of your workouts to note improvements, challenges, and how you feel after each session· Seeing your progress in black and white can be incredibly motivating and helps reinforce your commitment to the practice·

3· Stay Social: Exercising with friends or joining a class can enhance motivation· Consider inviting a friend to join you for Wall Pilates, or participate in community classes· The camaraderie will not only make it more fun but will also hold you accountable·

4· Celebrate Your Achievements: Celebrate your milestones, no matter how small! Whether it's mastering a new exercise or feeling more balanced, acknowledging your progress reinforces positive behavior and keeps you motivated·

5· Mix Things Up: Keep your workouts fresh by varying the exercises or trying new combinations· This can prevent boredom and stimulate your muscles in different ways·

6· Listen to Your Body: Pay attention to how your body feels during and after each workout· If something feels off or uncomfortable, don't hesitate to adjust your routine· Adapting to your body's signals helps maintain a positive experience and encourages a sustainable practice·

7· Practice Mindfulness: Incorporate mindfulness into your practice by focusing on your breath and being present during each movement· This connection not only enhances your workout but can also be a powerful stress-reliever·

Combining exercises for a full-body workout in Wall Pilates is an effective way to achieve your fitness goals while keeping your routine exciting and varied· With each session, you're investing in your strength, flexibility, and overall health· Remember to stay motivated, and most importantly, have fun.

CHAPTER 7

Special Considerations for Seniors

As we age, our bodies undergo various changes that may affect our strength, flexibility, and balance· Understanding these changes and tailoring our exercises to accommodate them is crucial for safe and effective practice· As your Wall Pilates coach, I want to guide you through these considerations, ensuring that you can enjoy the incredible benefits of Wall Pilates while prioritizing your health and safety·

The aging process brings unique challenges, but it also presents a wonderful opportunity to develop a deeper connection with your body· Recognizing and respecting your body's signals is key to enhancing your physical health and overall well-being·

Here's why special considerations are vital:

1. Our joints, muscles, and connective tissues can become more sensitive over time· By adapting exercises, we can reduce the risk of injury and ensure that every movement is safe and supportive·

2. As we age, maintaining mobility becomes increasingly important· Tailoring your Wall Pilates routine helps improve flexibility and joint health, making daily activities easier and more enjoyable·

3. Knowing that your workout is designed specifically for your needs can boost your confidence and encourage you to stay consistent· You'll feel empowered to take control of your health, one exercise at a time·

4. Balance is essential for preventing falls, which can be a significant concern for seniors· By focusing on exercises that enhance stability, you can improve your confidence in daily movements and maintain your independence·

What to Keep in Mind

Keep the following considerations in mind:

- **Consult Your Healthcare Provider:** Always check with your doctor before starting any new exercise program, especially if you have existing health conditions or concerns·
- **Listen to Your Body:** Pay attention to how your body responds to each exercise· It's perfectly okay to modify or skip certain movements if they don't feel right for you·
- **Start Slow and Progress Gradually:** Focus on mastering the basics before moving on to more challenging exercises· Gradual progression allows your body to adapt safely, minimizing the risk of injury·
- **Use Props for Support:** Don't hesitate to use supportive props like mats, pillows, or chairs· These can enhance your comfort and stability while performing various movements·
- **Focus on Breath and Mindfulness:** Breathing deeply and staying present

during your practice can enhance the benefits of each exercise· Mindfulness not only improves your physical performance but also promotes mental relaxation·

Wall Pilates is a powerful tool for maintaining and improving your strength, flexibility, and balance as you age· By understanding and implementing these special considerations, you can create a safe and effective practice that meets your unique needs· Remember, this journey is all about you, your progress, your comfort, and your health·

Addressing Common Health Issues

It's essential to understand how specific health issues can impact your practice and how we can adapt our exercises to accommodate those needs· Many seniors face health challenges that may affect their mobility, strength, or overall comfort during exercise· Here are some common health issues and how Wall Pilates can be adapted to support your needs:

Arthritis

Arthritis can lead to joint pain, stiffness, and reduced range of motion·

Adaptations: Focus on gentle movements that promote joint mobility without straining the affected areas· Incorporate exercises like Wall Roll Downs to gently stretch the spine and surrounding muscles· Always avoid any movements that cause discomfort, and work within a pain-free range·

Osteoporosis

Osteoporosis weakens bones, increasing the risk of fractures·

Adaptations: Prioritize low-impact exercises that strengthen muscles around the bones to enhance stability and support· Focus on exercises like Wall Squats and Wall Leg Lifts, which help improve muscle tone without putting excessive pressure on the spine· Avoid exercises that involve forward bending or twisting, as these can increase the risk of injury·

Balance Issues

Many seniors experience balance challenges, which can lead to falls·

Adaptations: Incorporate exercises that focus on stability and core strength, such as Wall Planks or Standing Leg Circles· Always keep a stable surface, like a wall or chair, nearby for support· Gradually increase the challenge by reducing your reliance on support as your balance improves·

Limited Flexibility

Aging can lead to decreased flexibility, making it harder to perform certain movements·

Adaptations: Integrate stretching-focused exercises like the Standing Roll Down and Wall Pike to enhance flexibility gently· Remember to breathe deeply and move slowly into each stretch, allowing your muscles to relax and lengthen·

Chronic Pain

Conditions like fibromyalgia or chronic pain syndromes can lead to discomfort during exercise·

Adaptations: Modify movements to accommodate comfort levels, starting with gentle, low-intensity exercises· Focus on breath control and mindfulness to help manage pain· Always listen to your body and adjust your routine as necessary·

Tips for Practicing Safely with Health Issues

- **Consult Your Healthcare Provider**: Always discuss your exercise plans with your doctor or physical therapist, especially if you have specific health concerns or are recovering from an injury·
- **Warm-Up and Cool Down:** Start each session with a gentle warm-up to prepare your muscles and joints, and end with a cool-down to help your body recover· This is especially important for those with chronic pain or stiffness·

- **Stay Hydrated:** Proper hydration is essential, particularly if you experience any medications that may affect your hydration levels· Drink water before, during, and after your workouts·

- **Use Supportive Props:** Use pillows, mats, or resistance bands to enhance comfort and support during your practice· These props can help make movements easier and more accessible·

- **Practice Mindfulness:** Pay attention to your body's signals and be mindful of how you feel during each exercise· If something doesn't feel right, it's okay to modify or skip that movement·

Addressing common health issues is a crucial aspect of your Wall Pilates journey· By understanding how these challenges can impact your practice and implementing appropriate adaptations, you can safely enjoy the many benefits of Wall Pilates· This practice is designed to enhance your strength, flexibility, and overall well-being while respecting your unique needs· You are in control of your body, and it's all about moving safely and effectively·

Modifying Exercises for Arthritis

Arthritis can make traditional exercises challenging, but with thoughtful modifications, you can enjoy the benefits of Wall Pilates safely and effectively· Arthritis is a condition characterized by inflammation of the joints, leading to pain, stiffness, and swelling· This can affect your range of motion and make certain movements uncomfortable· The good news is that Wall Pilates can be tailored to accommodate these challenges, allowing you to engage in physical activity that promotes joint health and mobility·

Key Modifications for Arthritis

1· Start with a gentle warm-up to increase blood flow to your joints and muscles· Try the following:

- Stand with your back against the wall and extend your arms out to the sides· Slowly make small circles in the air, gradually increasing the size· This movement warms up your shoulders without stressing your joints·

- While standing against the wall, gently roll your head in circles, moving from side to side· This helps to release tension in the neck and upper back·

2· Rather than a deep squat, slide down the wall only as far as comfortable· You can even use a chair behind you for additional support· Engage your core and keep your knees aligned over your ankles to avoid putting pressure on your joints·

3· Stand closer to the wall for a more upright push-up position· This reduces the load on your wrists and elbows· Keep your elbows slightly bent and your body in a straight line· Aim for 8-

10 repetitions, focusing on controlled movements·

4· Instead of lifting your leg high, lift it only to a level that feels comfortable· You can also perform the movement seated in a chair if standing is too challenging· Maintain a strong core and keep your standing leg slightly bent to reduce strain on your joints·

5· Sit on the floor with your back against the wall· Gently roll your spine down and then back up· This movement is less stressful on your joints while still promoting spinal mobility· Keep the movements slow and controlled, and breathe deeply to enhance relaxation·

6· End your practice with gentle stretches to promote relaxation and flexibility· Stand facing the wall, place your hands on it, and lean forward slightly to stretch your chest and shoulders· Stand facing the wall with one foot forward and press the back heel into the ground to stretch the calf.

Exercises for Improving Balance

By enhancing your balance, you can increase your confidence in daily activities and reduce the risk of falls· As we age, our balance can decline due to changes in muscle strength, coordination, and joint stability· Improved balance not only helps with mobility but also enhances your overall quality of life· With consistent practice, you can regain and maintain your stability, allowing you to move with ease and confidence·

Balance-Enhancing Exercises

1· **Wall Leg Lifts:** Stand facing the wall with your hands lightly resting on the surface for support· Lift one leg straight out to the side, keeping it aligned with your body· Hold for a few seconds, then lower it back down· Repeat 8-10 times on each side· Engage your core to maintain stability and avoid leaning toward the wall·

2· **Wall Single-Leg Balance:** Stand next to the wall and hold onto it for support· Lift one leg off the ground, bending the knee slightly· Hold this position for 10-30 seconds, then switch legs· Keep your standing leg slightly bent and engage your core to stay balanced·

3· Wall Heel Raises: Stand with your back against the wall and feet hip-width apart· Slowly raise your heels off the ground, balancing on your toes· Hold for a moment, then lower back down· Aim for 10-15 repetitions· Keep your core engaged and maintain a straight posture·

4· Wall Tai Chi Arm Movements: Stand facing the wall and extend your arms out to the sides at shoulder height· Slowly move your arms in a circular motion, simulating a Tai Chi movement· This helps improve coordination and balance while providing gentle support· Move fluidly and focus on your breath as you perform the movements·

5· Wall Marching: Stand facing the wall and hold on lightly· Begin marching in place, lifting your knees as high as comfortable· Start with 30 seconds, gradually increasing the time as you build strength and confidence· Keep your core engaged and focus on your posture throughout the exercise·

Incorporating modified exercises for arthritis and balance-enhancing movements into your Wall

Pilates practice will empower you to move confidently and comfortably· Every small step you take in your practice contributes to your overall well-being· Be patient with yourself, and celebrate your progress along the way·

Pilates for Osteoporosis

This condition requires special attention to ensure your bones stay protected while you build strength, balance, and flexibility· Osteoporosis is a condition that weakens bones, making them more fragile and prone to fractures· It's especially common in older adults, but the good news is that regular, mindful exercise can help improve bone density and reduce the risk of falls· Wall Pilates is an excellent choice because it offers gentle, low-impact movements that support bone health without putting undue strain on vulnerable areas· For those with osteoporosis, avoiding high-impact movements is key to preventing injury· Wall Pilates offers a safe, supportive environment where you can perform exercises with the assistance of the wall, helping you maintain balance and control while focusing on strengthening muscles that support your bones· By practicing these exercises regularly, you can improve your posture, enhance coordination, and build a stronger core, all while reducing the risk of fractures·

Key Pilates Principles for Osteoporosis

When practicing Wall Pilates with osteoporosis, we'll focus on three essential areas:

1. **Posture:** Good posture is vital to protecting your spine and bones· During each exercise, I'll guide you to align your body properly, lengthening your spine and engaging your core·
2. **Strength:** We'll focus on strengthening the muscles around your hips, spine, and legs, which support your bones and improve your balance·
3. **Flexibility:** Gentle stretching will help you maintain flexibility in your joints without stressing your bones· This enhances your

mobility and makes everyday movements easier·

Safe and Effective Exercises for Osteoporosis

Here are a few Wall Pilates exercises that are especially beneficial for those with osteoporosis:

Wall Squats:

How to Do It: Stand with your back against the wall, feet hip-width apart· Slowly slide down the wall into a shallow squat, keeping your knees aligned with your ankles· Hold for a few seconds, then press through your heels to stand back up·

Benefits: This strengthens the muscles around your hips and thighs, which helps support your bones· Keep the movement small and controlled to avoid straining your joints·

Wall Leg Lifts:

How to Do It: Stand next to the wall with one hand resting on it for support· Slowly lift one leg to the side, keeping it straight and your core engaged· Lower it back down and repeat 8-10 times before switching sides·

Benefits: This exercise strengthens your hip and leg muscles while improving balance, both of which are important for reducing the risk of falls·

Wall Planks:

How to Do It: Stand facing the wall, place your hands on it at shoulder height, and step your feet back slightly to create a plank position· Engage your core, keeping your body in a straight line· Hold for a few breaths, then release·

Benefits: This exercise engages your core and improves posture without putting pressure on your spine, making it ideal for those with osteoporosis·

Standing Roll Downs (Modified):

How to Do It: Stand tall with your back against the wall· Slowly roll down your spine, one vertebra at a time, only going as far as feels comfortable· Roll back up with control, engaging your core throughout·

Benefits: This gentle spinal movement helps increase flexibility and maintain mobility in your spine without forward flexion, which can be risky for individuals with osteoporosis·

Wall Heel Raises:

How to Do It: Stand with your back against the wall and feet hip-width apart· Slowly raise your heels off the ground, balancing on your toes· Hold for a moment, then lower back down· Repeat 10-15 times·

Benefits: This improves balance and strengthens your calves and ankles, which are important for stability and reducing fall risk·

Important Safety Tips

- **Avoid Forward Bending:** Exercises that involve bending forward from the waist, especially with a rounded back, can increase the risk of vertebral fractures·

Instead, focus on exercises that keep your spine long and neutral·

- **Move Slowly and Mindfully:** Always take your time during each exercise, moving with control· This helps prevent injuries and ensures you're engaging the correct muscles·

- **Focus on Core Strength:** A strong core supports your spine and improves your balance, both of which are essential for those with osteoporosis· Engage your core in every movement to protect your spine·

- **Use Props for Support:** Feel free to use a chair or any other prop for additional stability during exercises if needed·

Pilates for osteoporosis is about maintaining your bone health while strengthening the muscles that protect your body· These movements will not only help you feel stronger but also more confident in your daily activities· The wall is your friend—it's there to support and guide you through each movement·

CHAPTER 8

Incorporating Wall Pilates into Your Daily Activity

This chapter will guide you on effective movements that can be woven into your daily routine, helping you stay active and healthy without the need for a formal workout· Wall Pilates is not just something you do during a structured session; it's a practice that can support your well-being throughout the day· Whether you're brushing your teeth, standing in the kitchen, or even watching TV, the wall offers the perfect opportunity to sneak in some movement· The beauty of Wall Pilates is its versatility; you don't need fancy equipment, and you can do it anywhere there's a wall! Here, we'll explore how you can incorporate small but impactful exercises into everyday tasks· By making movement a natural part of your day, you'll improve your posture, strengthen your core, and enhance your flexibility—all while going about your regular activities· Plus, these small bursts of movement can help reduce stiffness and keep your joints mobile·

Integrating Exercises into Everyday Activities

Now that you've learned the foundations of Wall Pilates, let's take it a step further by incorporating these exercises into your daily routine· One of the best things about Wall Pilates is how adaptable it is to everyday life· You don't need a dedicated workout session to benefit from it—simple movements can be done throughout the day while you're standing, sitting, or even lying down·

As your Wall Pilates coach, I want you to think of movement as something you can weave seamlessly into your everyday tasks· Whether you're preparing a meal, watching TV, or waiting in line, you can engage your core, improve your posture, and stretch your muscles· These small, mindful actions will help you stay active, improve your flexibility, and build strength without feeling like you have to "make time" for exercise·

1· Wall Squats While Brushing Your Teeth

How to Do It: The next time you're brushing your teeth, try sliding down the wall into a wall squat· Stand with your back against the wall, feet hip-width apart, and slowly lower yourself into a squat position· Hold for the duration of brushing, then slowly stand back up·

Benefits: This strengthens your legs and core while improving balance and posture· Plus, it's a great way to make the most of those two minutes!

2· Standing Leg Lifts While Cooking

How to Do It: As you're waiting for water to boil or watching over a simmering pot, take a moment to do some standing leg lifts· Rest one hand on the kitchen counter for balance and lift one leg out to the side, keeping it straight· Lower it back down and repeat on the other side·

Benefits: This simple exercise strengthens your hips and improves your stability, which is essential for preventing falls·

3· Heel Raises While Waiting

How to Do It: Whether you're waiting in line or standing by the microwave, heel raises are an easy way to engage your calf muscles· Stand tall, hold onto a stable surface if needed, and slowly lift your heels off the ground· Hold for a second, then lower back down·

Benefits: Heel raises strengthen your calf muscles and improve ankle flexibility, which is great for better balance and foot mobility·

4· Wall Chest Stretch While Watching TV

How to Do It: As you watch your favorite show, take a moment to stretch out your chest· Stand facing the wall, place one hand on it at shoulder height, and gently rotate your body away from the wall until you feel a stretch in your chest and shoulder· Hold for 20-30 seconds, then switch sides·

Benefits: This stretch helps counteract the slouching that can happen when sitting, improving your posture and keeping your chest and shoulders open·

5· Seated Core Engagement While Sitting

How to Do It: Even while seated, you can engage your core and practice mindful posture· Sit up tall in your chair, roll your shoulders back, and gently pull your belly button toward your spine· Hold for a few seconds, then release· Repeat several times while sitting at the table or watching TV·

Benefits: This strengthens your core muscles and encourages good posture, which helps support your spine and overall stability·

6· Wall Push-Ups While Doing Household Chores

How to Do It: Take a break from folding laundry or tidying up to do a few wall push-ups· Place your hands on the wall at shoulder height, step your feet back, and lower your chest toward the wall, then press back up· Aim for 10-15 repetitions·

Benefits: Wall push-ups strengthen your upper body and core while being gentle on your joints· Plus, it's a great way to get a quick upper-body workout without going to the floor·

7· Wall Side Stretches After Gardening

How to Do It: After spending time in the garden or doing yard work, it's important to stretch out those tired muscles· Stand tall, place one hand on the wall, and reach the other arm overhead· Gently lean to the side, feeling a stretch along your side and rib cage· Hold for a few breaths, then switch sides·

Benefits: This stretch helps release tension in your sides and lower back, improving flexibility and range of motion·

Incorporating Wall Pilates into your daily routine doesn't have to be complicated· By adding these simple exercises and stretches into your everyday activities, you'll find it easier to stay active, improve your posture, and strengthen your muscles· These movements may be small, but they add up over time, contributing to your overall health and well-being· Remember, the key to success is consistency· Make movement a natural part of your day, and you'll start to feel the benefits in your body—more strength, more balance, and more flexibility· With every mindful movement, you're investing in a healthier, more vibrant version of yourself!

Simple Stretching Routines

Stretching is an essential part of keeping your body mobile, flexible, and ready for movement· Stretching not only helps prevent stiffness, but it also improves your range of motion and supports joint health· Plus, with Wall Pilates, the wall is your steady companion, giving you the support you need to stretch safely and confidently·

Here are a few simple stretches you can do throughout the day to keep your body feeling its best:

1· Wall Chest Opener
How to Do It: Stand about a foot away from the wall, place one hand on it at shoulder height, and gently turn your body away from the wall· Hold the stretch for 20-30 seconds, then switch sides·
Benefits: This stretch helps open up the chest, improve posture, and release tension in your shoulders, which is especially helpful if you spend a lot of time sitting·
2· Standing Hamstring Stretch

How to Do It: Face the wall, place your hands on it for support, and step one leg forward with the other leg extended straight behind you· Slowly lean forward over your front leg, keeping your back straight and your hips level· Hold for 20-30 seconds, then switch legs·

Benefits: This stretch targets the hamstrings and lower back, helping to relieve tightness and improve flexibility in your legs·

3· Side Body Stretch

How to Do It: Stand with your side next to the wall, place one hand on the wall for support, and reach your other arm up and over your head, gently stretching your side· Hold for 20-30 seconds, then switch sides·

Benefits: This stretch lengthens the muscles along your sides and rib cage, increasing flexibility and improving your range of motion, especially around the waist and back·

4· Wall Calf Stretch

How to Do It: Stand facing the wall, place both hands on it, and step one foot back while keeping it flat on the ground· Lean into the wall to stretch the back leg's calf· Hold for 20-30 seconds, then switch legs·

Benefits: This stretch helps loosen up tight calf muscles and improves ankle flexibility, which is important for maintaining balance and mobility·

5· Standing Quadriceps Stretch

How to Do It: Stand facing the wall, place one hand on it for balance, and grab your opposite ankle behind you· Gently pull your heel toward your buttock, feeling a stretch in the front of your thigh· Hold for 20-30 seconds, then switch legs·

Benefits: This stretch helps relieve tension in the quadriceps and improves flexibility in your thighs, which is key for supporting knee and hip joints·

Tips for Effective Stretching

- As you stretch, focus on slow, deep breaths· Inhale deeply to expand your lungs, and exhale as you gently ease into the stretch· This helps your muscles relax and improves circulation·

- Never force a stretch· Move slowly and stop if you feel any pain· The goal is to gently lengthen your muscles, not to push them beyond their limits·
- Aim to hold each stretch for 20-30 seconds, allowing your muscles time to release tension and fully stretch out·
- Try doing these stretches at least once a day, whether it's in the morning to wake up your muscles or in the evening to wind down and relax·

These simple stretches are a great way to keep your body limber and energized throughout the day· By taking just a few minutes to stretch regularly, you'll notice improvements in your flexibility, posture, and overall comfort· Stretching is one of the easiest things you can do to support your body, and with the wall as your guide, it's accessible to everyone—no matter your fitness level·

Quick Workouts for Busy Days

Life can get busy, but that doesn't mean you need to skip out on keeping your body active! In this Quick Workouts for Busy Days section, I'll show you how to stay consistent with your Wall Pilates practice even on those hectic days·   These mini-workouts are designed to target key areas of your body, improve flexibility, and keep your muscles engaged—all in just a few minutes· You don't need a long session to reap the benefits of Pilates; it's all about quality movements· The great thing about Wall Pilates is that you can perform these exercises at any time, anywhere there's a wall·

1· Wall Plank (1 minute)

How to Do It: Stand facing the wall, place your hands on the wall at shoulder height, and step your feet back until your body forms a straight line from head to heels· Hold this position for 30 seconds to 1 minute, engaging your core and maintaining a straight spine·

Benefits: The wall plank strengthens your core, arms, and shoulders, giving you a full-body workout in just a minute·

2· Wall Squats (2 minutes)

How to Do It: Stand with your back against the wall, feet hip-width apart, and slowly slide down the wall until your thighs are parallel to the floor· Hold for 30 seconds, stand back up, and repeat for 2 minutes·

Benefits: Wall squats work your legs, glutes, and core while improving your balance and stability·

3· Wall Push-Ups (2 minutes)

How to Do It: Stand facing the wall, place your hands on it at shoulder height, and step back slightly· Slowly lower your chest toward the wall, then push back to the starting position· Repeat for 1-2 minutes·

Benefits: Wall push-ups are an excellent way to build upper body strength in your chest, shoulders, and arms without putting too much pressure on your joints·

4· Standing Side Leg Lifts (2 minutes)

How to Do It: Stand next to the wall, using one hand for balance· Lift one leg out to the side, keeping it straight, then slowly lower it back down· Repeat for 1 minute on each side·

Benefits: This exercise strengthens the outer hips and improves balance, which is crucial for fall prevention·

5· Seated Wall Roll Down (2 minutes)

How to Do It: Sit tall with your back against the wall, feet flat on the floor· Slowly roll your spine away from the wall, lowering your upper body toward your knees while engaging your core· Hold for a moment, then slowly roll back up to the starting position· Repeat for 2 minutes·

Benefits: This movement engages your core and stretches your spine, promoting flexibility and posture·

Tips for Quick Workouts

- Even in a short workout, proper form is key· Pay attention to your alignment and engage your muscles with intention·
- These quick routines are designed to be done in 5-10 minutes, so try to fit them in whenever you have a few spare moments·

Consistency, even in small doses, will make a big difference over time·

- Remember to breathe deeply throughout your exercises· Inhale to prepare, and exhale as you perform each movement· This helps you stay calm and focused while working out·

When life gets busy, it's easy to put exercise on the back burner, but Wall Pilates offers a flexible way to keep moving, no matter how tight your schedule is· These quick, efficient routines are perfect for squeezing in movement during breaks, before bed, or anytime you have a few free minutes· Even on your busiest days, a few minutes of Pilates can help you stay strong, mobile, and energized· The key is to keep moving consistency, even in small doses, will help you stay on track with your fitness goals·

Tracking Your Progress

Keeping track of your Wall Pilates journey is not just about celebrating your improvements it's also a powerful motivator to stay consistent· Progress in Pilates isn't just about being able to do more repetitions or holding positions longer (although that's certainly part of it)· It's also about how you feel your flexibility, posture, balance, and overall comfort in daily activities· Wall Pilates is designed to improve your quality of life, and tracking your progress will allow you to see the benefits over time·

Why Tracking is Important

- Seeing your improvements, no matter how small, keeps you motivated and boosts your confidence· Tracking lets you recognize your hard work·

- It helps you stay mindful of your body· You'll notice which exercises get easier and where you might need to focus more attention·

- Tracking gives you a clear picture of your starting point and where you want to go· Whether it's improving flexibility, increasing strength, or maintaining a daily routine, tracking helps you set realistic and achievable goals·

Ways to Track Your Progress

- After each workout, jot down what you did, how you felt, and any changes you notice· You can note the number of repetitions, how long you held a position, or even how your balance or flexibility improved· Over time, this journal becomes a great record of your achievements·
- Every month, take a few minutes to assess your strength and flexibility· Measure how far you can reach in a stretch or how long you can hold a Wall Plank or Wall Squat· Write down the results to compare them to previous months·
- Pay attention to how your body feels during and after workouts· Do you feel less stiff when you wake up? Are you able to sit or stand more comfortably? These are signs of progress that you might not always see on paper, but they're just as important·

- Progress is progress, no matter the size· Did you add a few extra seconds to your Wall Plank? That's worth celebrating! These small milestones build the foundation for long-term success·

What to Look for as You Progress
- Notice how much easier it becomes to perform certain stretches or how much deeper you can go into a stretch without discomfort·
- As your core and back muscles strengthen, you might notice yourself standing taller or sitting with more ease·
- Are you feeling steadier on your feet? This is a great indicator of improvement in your strength and stability·
- Pay attention to how much easier it is to perform exercises like Wall Push-Ups or Wall Squats compared to when you first started·

Tracking your progress is all about recognizing the small victories along the way· Wall Pilates is a journey, and each step, no matter how small, gets you closer to your goals· By keeping a record of how far you've come, you can see the real changes happening in your body and your health· Plus, it gives you the extra motivation to stay consistent with your practice· Remember, the progress you make is unique to you· Whether it's gaining flexibility, feeling stronger, or just staying active, your journey is worth celebrating· So, grab a notebook, track those milestones, and let's keep moving forward together!

CHAPTER 9

Nutrition and Recovery

I want to emphasize that exercise is only one part of the equation for staying healthy and active· Proper nutrition and recovery are equally important, especially for seniors· Together, they fuel your body, support muscle growth, and ensure that you're ready for your next workout· Recovery doesn't just mean resting after your Wall Pilates session—it's about giving your body the nutrients it needs to repair and recharge· In this chapter, we'll explore how smart nutrition choices can aid in your recovery, enhance your performance, and improve your overall well-being· The right balance of foods, along with proper hydration, helps maintain strong muscles, flexible joints, and stable energy levels· Let's start with how you can fuel your body and make the most of your Wall Pilates practice, both on and off the mat!

Importance of Nutrition for Seniors

Your body is like a finely tuned machine especially as you get older, it needs the right fuel to keep it running smoothly· While Wall Pilates is fantastic for building strength, flexibility, and balance, what you eat plays an equally critical role in supporting your fitness journey· Proper nutrition helps your body recover from exercise, maintain muscle mass, and keep your energy levels up, ensuring you stay active and strong for years to come· As we age, our nutritional needs change· You may require fewer calories, but your body still needs the same, if not more, nutrients to stay healthy· Seniors often face a reduction in muscle mass, bone density, and metabolism, which makes focusing on nutrient-rich foods even more crucial· By making mindful food choices, you can maintain the strength and vitality necessary for your Wall Pilates practice and your everyday life·

Key Nutrients for Seniors

Protein: Think of protein as the building block for your muscles· After each Wall Pilates session, your muscles need protein to repair and grow stronger· Include lean protein sources like chicken, turkey, fish, eggs, beans, and tofu in your meals· Aim for small but consistent servings of protein throughout the day to keep your muscles nourished·

Calcium and Vitamin D: These are essential for maintaining strong bones· Weight-bearing exercises like Wall Squats help strengthen bones, but calcium and vitamin D are the nutrients that support bone density· Include foods like dairy products, leafy greens, and fortified foods in your diet, and get plenty of sunlight for that vitamin D boost!

Healthy Fats: Omega-3 fatty acids found in fish, walnuts, and flaxseeds are important for reducing inflammation, which can ease joint pain and stiffness—especially helpful after a workout· Healthy fats also help support brain health and overall well-being·

Fiber: As we age, digestion can slow down, and fiber becomes crucial for maintaining healthy digestion and preventing constipation· Whole grains, fruits, vegetables, and legumes are great sources of fiber that will also provide you with sustained energy for your workouts·

Hydration: Staying hydrated is vital, especially when you're active· Water keeps your joints lubricated, helps with muscle recovery, and supports overall body function· Make it a habit to drink water throughout the day, not just when you're thirsty·

Pre- and Post-Workout Nutrition

Have a light snack that combines complex carbohydrates and a bit of protein· Something like a piece of fruit with a handful of nuts or yogurt with berries will give you the energy to power through your Wall Pilates routine without weighing you down· Refueling after your session is key to recovery· A balanced meal with protein, healthy fats, and complex carbohydrates will help your muscles recover and give you lasting energy· A good example would be grilled chicken with quinoa and steamed vegetables or a smoothie with protein powder, spinach, and almond milk·

Nutrition works hand-in-hand with recovery· After your Wall Pilates workout, your body needs time to repair and rebuild· Sleep is a huge part of this, but so is nourishing your body with the right foods· Incorporating anti-inflammatory foods—like berries, leafy greens, and nuts—can help speed up recovery and reduce soreness, allowing you to stay consistent with your practice· Proper nutrition is like the engine behind your Wall Pilates routine· It supports muscle recovery, maintains energy, and helps you stay agile and strong as you age· By focusing on nutrient-dense foods and staying hydrated, you'll maximize the benefits of your Wall Pilates sessions and keep your body feeling its best· So, as you continue with your workouts, remember: what you put on your plate is just as important as the time you spend at the wall·

Hydration Tips

Proper hydration is crucial for getting the most out of your workouts, especially as you age· Staying hydrated is essential for muscle function, joint health, and overall energy levels· Water is essential for nearly every function in the body· It helps regulate body temperature, lubricate joints, transport nutrients, and remove waste· During exercise, your body loses water through sweat, even if you're not sweating heavily· If you're dehydrated, your muscles may cramp, and your joints can feel stiff, making it harder to move smoothly through your Pilates exercises·

As we age, our sense of thirst can decrease, making it easier to become dehydrated without realizing it· That's why it's even more important to make a conscious effort to stay hydrated·

Hydration Tips for Seniors
Drink Consistently Throughout the Day

Don't wait until you're thirsty to drink water· Sip water regularly throughout the day to keep your body well-hydrated· Aim for 6-8 glasses of water daily, but listen to your body's needs, especially when exercising·

Hydrate Before and After Workouts
It's important to start your Wall Pilates session well-hydrated· Drink a glass of water about 30 minutes before you begin your workout· After your session, rehydrate by drinking water to replace any fluids lost during exercise·

Flavor Your Water
If you find plain water boring, try adding slices of lemon, cucumber, or fresh mint to your water for a refreshing twist· Herbal teas or infused water can also help make hydration more enjoyable without adding sugars·

Pay Attention to Your Body's Signals
Signs of dehydration can include feeling tired, dizzy, or having a dry mouth· If you notice these signs during or after your Wall Pilates practice, it's time to take a break and hydrate· Dark-colored urine is another indicator that you may need to drink more water·

Carry a Water Bottle

Keep a water bottle nearby when doing your Wall Pilates exercises· This simple habit ensures you can take small sips during your routine without interrupting your flow· If you have limited mobility, position your water bottle where it's easy to reach between exercises·

Incorporate Hydrating Foods

In addition to drinking water, you can stay hydrated by incorporating water-rich foods like fruits and vegetables into your diet· Foods like cucumbers, watermelon, oranges, and leafy greens contain high water content and provide essential vitamins and minerals·

Monitor Your Caffeine and Alcohol Intake

Caffeine and alcohol can act as diuretics, meaning they may lead to increased water loss· If you enjoy tea, coffee, or a glass of wine, make sure to balance it out with extra water to stay hydrated·

Hydration is key to helping your body perform at its best—both during and after your Wall Pilates workouts· Keeping yourself hydrated ensures that your muscles work efficiently, your joints remain flexible, and your energy stays steady throughout the day· Remember, hydration is not just about quenching your thirst; it's about caring for your body's needs as you work toward improved health and fitness· So, grab your water bottle, drink up, and let's keep moving!

Post-Workout Recovery Strategies

Congratulations on completing your Wall Pilates session! Now, let's talk about one of the most important parts of your exercise routine recovery· Effective recovery helps your body rebuild, recharge, and get ready for your next session· It can prevent injuries, reduce soreness, and enhance your overall performance·

During your Wall Pilates workout, your muscles work hard to support your movements· The small tears that occur in your muscles need time to repair, which is where recovery comes in· With proper recovery, your muscles heal stronger, your flexibility improves, and your overall stamina increases· For seniors, this is especially important to maintain mobility and prevent strain or injury·

Key Post-Workout Recovery Strategies

- After a workout, your muscles are warm and more flexible· Take advantage of this by spending a few minutes gently stretching the areas you've worked· This helps to increase blood flow, which speeds up recovery and reduces soreness· Incorporate slow, deep breathing as you stretch to relax both your body and mind·
- Hydration is a vital part of recovery· After exercising, your body needs to replenish the fluids lost through sweat· Drinking water after your session helps flush out toxins, aids in muscle recovery, and prevents cramping· Add a slice of lemon or cucumber to your water for a refreshing post-workout drink·
- Eating a light snack within 30 minutes after your Wall Pilates session can aid in muscle

repair· A combination of protein and carbohydrates helps rebuild muscle fibers and restores energy· Consider a snack like Greek yogurt with fruit, a protein smoothie, or a small handful of nuts and a banana·

- Using a foam roller or even your hands to gently massage your muscles can help relieve tension and improve circulation· A few minutes of self-massage on your legs, back, or arms can reduce stiffness and make your muscles feel more relaxed·

- Your body does most of its recovery work while you sleep· Aim for 7-9 hours of quality sleep each night to allow your muscles and joints to fully recover· Rest is the time when your body repairs and strengthens itself, ensuring you're ready for your next Wall Pilates session·

- Recovery isn't just about taking a break; it's about being in tune with your body· Pay attention to how you feel after your workout· If you're experiencing discomfort or fatigue, it may be a sign that you need to rest longer, stretch more, or modify your exercises· Remember, consistency is important, but so is giving your body the time it needs to heal·

- Not every day needs to be a full workout day· On your recovery days, try light activities like walking, swimming, or gentle stretching to keep your body moving without over-exertion· Active recovery helps reduce stiffness and keeps your joints limber without putting too much strain on your muscles·

Recovery is your body's way of saying, "Thank you" for all the hard work you've done· It's an essential part of maintaining strength, flexibility, and overall well-being, especially as you get older· By following these recovery strategies, you'll help your body repair and rejuvenate, so you're always feeling ready for the next Wall Pilates session· Remember, recovery isn't a break from progress it's part of the journey·

Sample Meal Plans

Proper nutrition fuels not just your workouts but your overall well-being· What you eat before and after exercise plays a critical role in supporting your strength, flexibility, and recovery· These sample meal plans are designed to help you get the right balance of nutrients, ensuring your body stays energized and nourished throughout your Wall Pilates journey· The goal is to provide meals that are easy to prepare, nutrient-dense, and perfectly suited for seniors looking to maintain muscle mass, bone health, and energy levels· Whether you're a beginner or have been practicing for a while, these meal plans will help you feel your best both in and out of your Pilates routine·

Meal Plan 1

On days when your Wall Pilates session is lighter or you're focusing on stretching, you'll want meals that keep you satisfied without feeling too heavy·

Breakfast

Oatmeal with Fresh Berries and Almonds

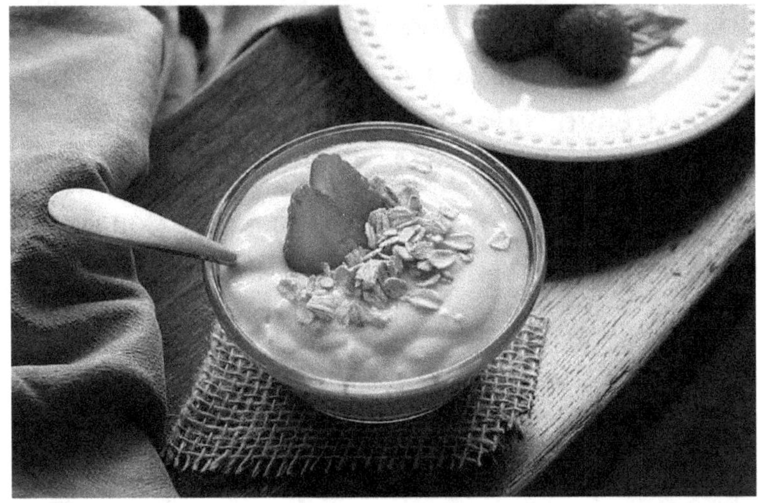

Start your day with a bowl of warm oatmeal, topped with antioxidant-rich berries and a sprinkle of heart-healthy almonds· Oats provide long-lasting energy, while the berries add a burst of flavor and vitamins·

Tip: Add a dash of cinnamon for extra anti-inflammatory benefits·

Lunch

Spinach Salad with Grilled Chicken and Avocado

This light yet nourishing salad combines protein from lean grilled chicken with the healthy fats in avocado· The spinach provides iron, which helps keep you feeling strong, while the avocado keeps your joints lubricated·

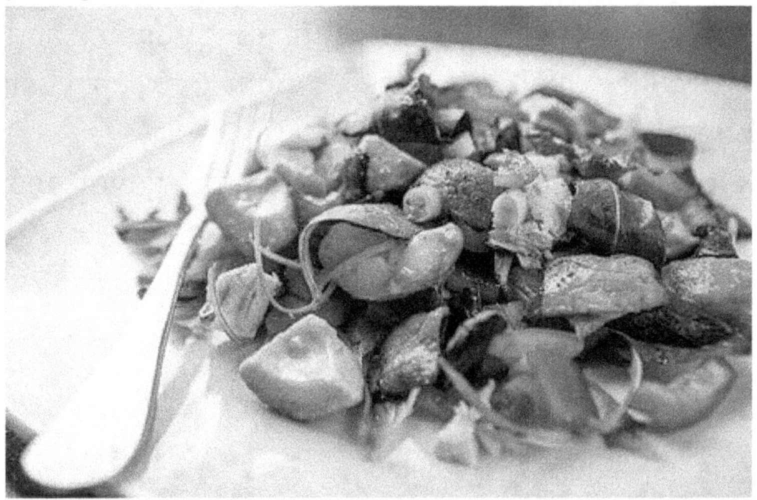

Tip: Drizzle with olive oil and lemon for a simple, flavorful dressing·

Snack

Greek Yogurt with Honey and Walnuts
Greek yogurt is high in protein and perfect for muscle recovery· Add a touch of honey for sweetness and walnuts for a dose of omega-3 fatty acids to reduce inflammation·

Dinner

Baked Salmon with Quinoa and Steamed Broccoli
Salmon is rich in omega-3s, which support heart health and reduce inflammation· Pair it with quinoa, a whole grain full of protein, and broccoli, which provides calcium to keep your bones strong·

Tip: Add garlic and herbs for extra flavor and antioxidants·

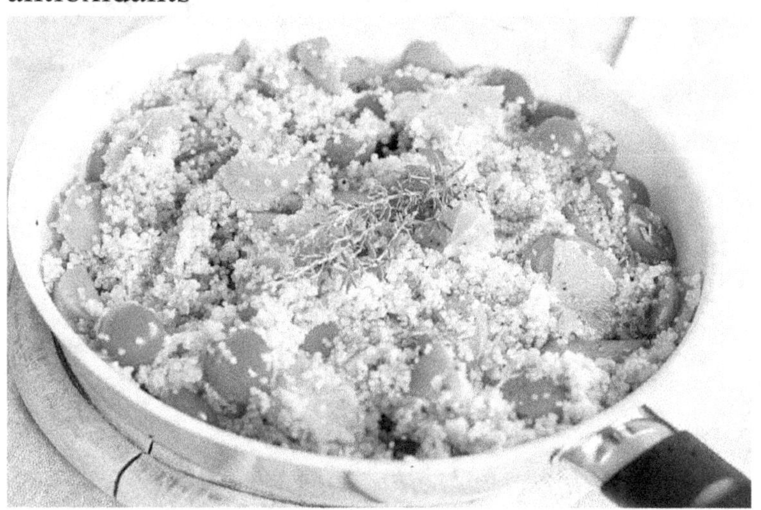

Meal Plan 2: For More Intense Workout Days

On days when you're tackling more challenging Wall Pilates exercises, your meals should focus on replenishing your energy and aiding muscle recovery·

Breakfast

Scrambled Eggs with Whole Grain Toast and Sautéed Spinach

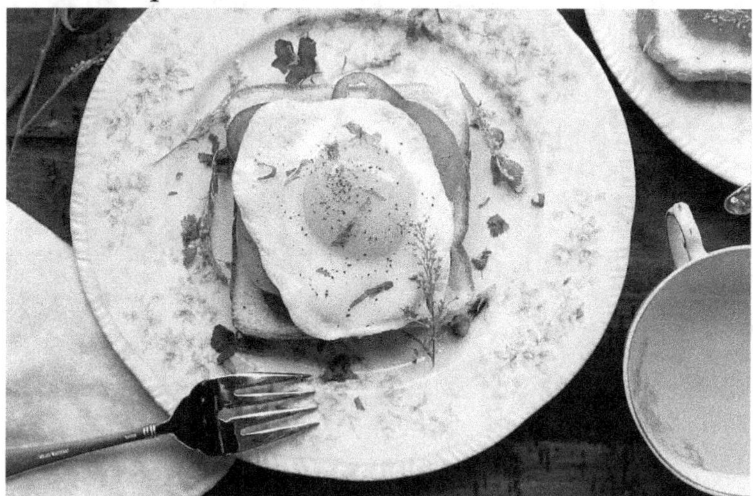

Eggs are packed with protein, which is essential for repairing muscles after exercise· The whole grain toast provides slow-releasing carbohydrates, and spinach adds a boost of iron and fiber·

Tip: Sauté your spinach in olive oil for added healthy fats·

Lunch

Quinoa and Chickpea Power Bowl with Mixed Vegetables

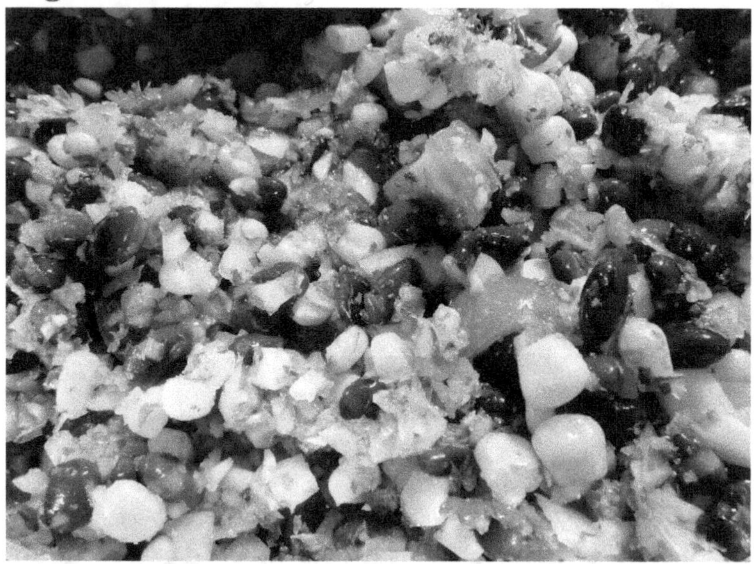

This plant-based lunch is a powerhouse of protein, fiber, and vitamins· Quinoa and chickpeas are both excellent sources of protein, while the colorful vegetables offer a variety of nutrients·

Tip: Add a spoonful of hummus or tahini for extra flavor and creamy texture·

Snack

Apple Slices with Almond Butter

A simple but effective snack to boost energy and keep hunger at bay· Apples provide fiber and natural sugars, while almond butter is rich in healthy fats and protein·

Dinner

Turkey Stir-Fry with Brown Rice and Vegetables

Lean turkey is great for muscle repair after a more intense workout· Brown rice provides complex carbohydrates to restore energy, while the veggies (carrots, bell peppers, zucchini) add color and essential vitamins·

Tip: Use a low-sodium soy sauce or coconut aminos for a healthier stir-fry·

Meal Plan 3: Recovery and Rest Day

On your rest or recovery days, it's important to continue nourishing your body with meals that are gentle but nutrient-rich·

Breakfast

Chia Seed Pudding with Almond Milk and Blueberries

Chia seeds are rich in omega-3s and fiber, which help reduce inflammation and keep digestion running smoothly· Almond milk provides calcium, and blueberries give a dose of antioxidants·

Tip: Prepare this the night before for a quick and easy breakfast·

Lunch

Lentil Soup with Whole Grain Crackers

Lentils are an excellent plant-based protein, perfect for muscle repair· The soup is warming and easy to digest, while whole grain crackers provide fiber and additional energy·

Tip: Add a handful of fresh herbs like parsley for extra nutrients and flavor·

Snack

Cottage Cheese with Pineapple

Cottage cheese is high in protein, and the natural sweetness of pineapple adds a refreshing burst of vitamin C· This snack is great for helping your muscles recover and keeping your bones strong·

Dinner

Grilled Chicken with Sweet Potato and Green Beans

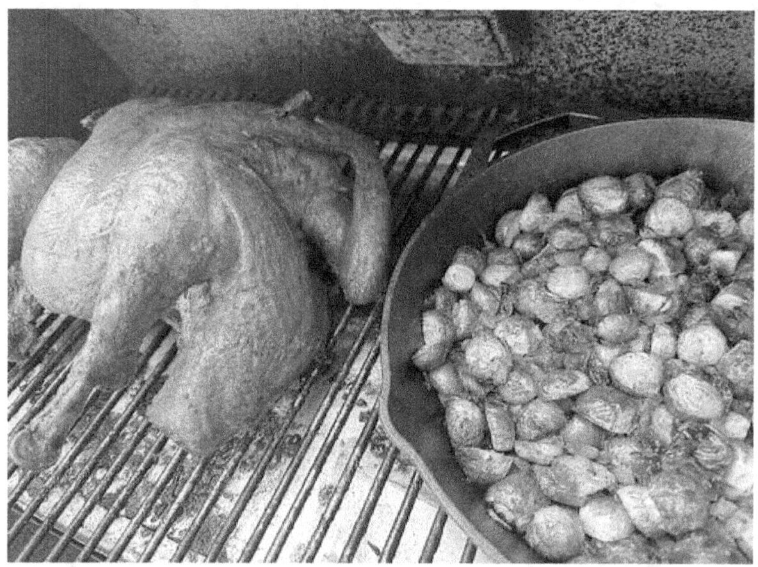

Sweet potatoes are full of complex carbohydrates and fiber, while green beans offer a good dose of vitamins A and C· Grilled chicken provides lean protein to keep your muscles healthy and strong·
Tip: Bake the sweet potatoes with a little olive oil and cinnamon for added flavor and anti-inflammatory properties·

These sample meal plans are designed to complement your Wall Pilates practice by fueling your body with the right nutrients· By incorporating balanced meals rich in protein, healthy fats, fiber, and essential vitamins and minerals, you'll not only enhance your performance during Pilates but also support recovery, improve energy levels, and maintain overall health· Remember, food is fuel· Eat mindfully, stay hydrated, and listen to your body's needs·

CHAPTER 10

Frequently Asked Questions

I understand that you may have questions or concerns· This section aims to address the most common questions from seniors just like you, which may help to clarify any uncertainties and ensure you feel confident in your practice· You may be curious about what to expect in your practice, how to get started, or how to adapt exercises for your specific fitness level· Maybe you're wondering how often you should practice or what to wear· Whatever your questions may be, I'm here to guide you through them·

Common Concerns and Solutions

This section addresses some common questions and provides practical solutions to help you feel confident and safe as you embark on your Wall Pilates journey·

I'm New to Exercise· Is Wall Pilates Right for Me?

Solution: Absolutely! Wall Pilates is an excellent choice for beginners, especially seniors· The wall provides stability and support, making it easier to maintain balance and proper form· Start with basic exercises and gradually progress to more challenging movements as you become more comfortable· Always listen to your body and take breaks as needed·

I Have Limited Mobility or Joint Pain· Can I Still Participate?

Solution: Yes, you can! Wall Pilates is highly adaptable, and many exercises can be modified to suit your mobility level· Use the wall for support, and don't hesitate to make adjustments to reduce strain on your joints· It's essential to consult your doctor or physical therapist before starting any new exercise program, especially if you have existing conditions· They can provide guidance on which exercises are best for you·

I'm Afraid I Might Fall·

Solution: Safety is our top priority· The wall is a great support system, helping you maintain balance during exercises· Start with exercises that are low to the ground and gradually incorporate movements that challenge your stability· Always work in a safe, clutter-free area, and consider having a friend or family member nearby until you feel more confident·

I Don't Have the Right Equipment·
Solution: One of the best aspects of Wall Pilates is that it requires minimal equipment· All you need is a wall, a comfortable mat, and possibly some lightweight resistance bands or a small ball for added support and challenge· If you don't have access to these, don't worry! Many exercises can be performed with just your body weight and the wall·

I'm Not Flexible· Will I Be Able to Do Wall Pilates?
Solution: Flexibility comes with practice! Wall Pilates can help improve your flexibility over time· Start with gentle stretches and focus on

maintaining good form rather than pushing yourself too hard· As you practice regularly, you'll notice gradual improvements in your flexibility and overall range of motion·

I'm Not Sure How to Breathe Properly During Exercises·

Solution: Breathing is a crucial part of Pilates! Focus on inhaling through your nose as you prepare for a movement and exhaling through your mouth as you execute the movement· Think of your breath as a way to fuel your movements, helping you to engage your core and maintain control· If you're unsure, practice breathing exercises on their own before incorporating them into your workouts·

I Might Get Tired or Overwhelmed·

Solution: It's perfectly normal to feel tired, especially if you're new to exercise· Listen to your body and take breaks as needed· Start with shorter sessions (10-15 minutes) and gradually increase the duration as your endurance improves· Remember, it's not about how much you do; it's about how consistently you practice·

How Often Should I Practice Wall Pilates?

Solution: Aim for at least 2-3 sessions per week to reap the benefits of Wall Pilates· Consistency is key! However, listen to your body; if you feel fatigued, allow yourself some rest days· You can also incorporate gentle stretches or active recovery days, like walking, to keep your body moving·

Addressing Myths about Pilates

Pilates is Only for Young People or Athletes·

<u>**Truth:**</u> Pilates is for everyone, regardless of age or fitness level! In fact, Wall Pilates is specifically designed to be gentle and supportive, making it an excellent choice for seniors· The exercises can be modified to suit individual needs, allowing you to strengthen your body at your own pace· Many older adults find that Pilates helps improve their strength, flexibility, and overall mobility·

You Need to Be Flexible to Do Pilates·
Truth: Flexibility is a benefit of practicing Pilates, not a prerequisite· Many seniors come to Wall Pilates with varying levels of flexibility, and that's perfectly okay! The wall provides stability and support, allowing you to perform movements safely and effectively· With regular practice, you'll gradually improve your flexibility and range of motion·

Pilates is Just About Abs·
Truth: While Pilates does focus on core strength, it encompasses much more than that· Wall Pilates engages multiple muscle groups, including your arms, legs, and back· It promotes overall body awareness, strength, and alignment, making it a comprehensive workout for all parts of your body·

Pilates is Too Easy and Doesn't Provide a Good Workout·
Truth: Pilates is not about how hard you push yourself; it's about the quality of your movements· Wall Pilates offers various levels of

intensity, and with the right modifications, it can be very challenging· The beauty of Pilates lies in its emphasis on control, precision, and breath, which can lead to significant improvements in strength and endurance over time·

You Need Special Equipment for Pilates·
Truth: While traditional Pilates may involve specialized equipment, Wall Pilates primarily utilizes a wall and your body weight· This makes it accessible to everyone, as you can easily practice in your home or anywhere with a wall· If you want to enhance your practice, a few lightweight resistance bands or a small ball can be helpful, but they are not necessary to get started·

Pilates is Not Suitable for Seniors with Health Conditions·
Truth: Wall Pilates can be beneficial for seniors with various health conditions, provided you have clearance from your healthcare provider· Many exercises can be modified to accommodate specific needs, such as joint pain, arthritis, or limited mobility· Always listen to your body and

consult with your doctor or physical therapist if you have any concerns before starting your practice·

You Have to Attend Classes to Learn Pilates·
<u>Truth:</u> While classes can be beneficial, you don't have to attend in-person sessions to learn Pilates· This book serves as a comprehensive guide, allowing you to follow along at your own pace in the comfort of your home· With clear instructions and visual aids, you can effectively practice Wall Pilates independently·

Resources for Further Learning

I believe that continuous learning is key to enhancing your practice and enjoying the many benefits of Pilates· Below, I've compiled a variety of resources that can help you deepen your understanding, refine your techniques, and stay motivated on your Wall Pilates journey·

Books

- "Pilates for Life" by Rachael O'Meara
- "The Pilates Body" by Brooke Siler
- "Strong Bones, Strong Body: Pilates for Seniors" by Janice M· Roebuck
- Wall Pilates Workouts for Women by Sophy Harrington
- The Comprehensive Guide to Wall Pilates for Seniors by Katherine Harmeen

Websites

- The Pilates Method Alliance (PMA): https://www.pilatesmethodalliance.org
- National Osteoporosis Foundation: https://www.bonehealthandosteoporosis.or
- Local Classes and Workshops

Conclusion

Throughout this book, we've explored various Wall Pilates exercises designed specifically for seniors, focusing on improving strength, flexibility, balance, and overall well-being· Each exercise is not just a movement but a step towards enhancing your quality of life· You've learned how to use the wall as a supportive tool, allowing you to perform exercises safely and effectively· This unique approach helps to reduce the risk of injury while promoting proper alignment and form· As you incorporate Wall Pilates into your routine, remember that consistency is key· Just as you've developed your skills through practice, you'll continue to grow stronger and more confident with each session· Listen to your body, and honor its needs· Some days, you may feel energized and ready to push your limits, while other days may call for gentler movements· Both are perfectly valid·

Wall Pilates utilizes the wall as a supportive tool, making it accessible and safe for seniors· It promotes stability and alignment, allowing you to perform exercises with confidence·

Targeted exercises help build core, upper, and lower body strength· Regular practice increases flexibility and range of motion in the joints· Wall Pilates focuses on improving balance and coordination, which is crucial for fall prevention· Engaging with your body through Pilates encourages mindfulness and enhances overall body awareness·

Key Exercises

Wall Squats: Strengthen the legs and improve stability·

Standing Roll Down: Enhance spinal flexibility and posture·

Wall Push-Ups: Build upper body strength while maintaining safety·

Wall Leg Lifts: Strengthen the hips and improve core stability·

It's normal to face challenges along the way, but don't let them discourage you· Every expert was once a beginner, and every journey has its ups and downs· Listen to your body, honor its limits, and celebrate your progress, no matter how minor it may seem· The key is consistency and patience; with each practice, you are laying the foundation for lasting benefits· Connect with others on this journey· Sharing your experiences with friends, family, or a supportive community can provide motivation and encouragement· You are not alone in this; many others are seeking the same growth and improvement· Above all, approach your Wall Pilates practice with a sense of curiosity and joy· Explore new exercises, try different variations, and discover what feels good for your body· This practice is not just about fitness; it's about nurturing your spirit and finding pleasure in movement· So, take a deep breath and embrace the journey ahead· Your commitment to Wall Pilates is a commitment to your health, vitality, and overall happiness· Remember, every moment spent moving, breathing, and connecting with your body is a valuable investment in your future·

In all, staying active is not just about physical exercise; it's about nurturing your overall well-being, fostering independence, and embracing a vibrant lifestyle· Wall Pilates offers a gentle yet effective way to engage your body, enhance your strength, flexibility, and balance, and promote a sense of vitality and joy in your daily life· As you incorporate Wall Pilates into your routine, remember that every small effort counts· Consistency is key, and even short, focused sessions can yield significant benefits over time· Celebrate the progress you make, whether it's increased flexibility, improved balance, or simply feeling more energized throughout the day· Each step you take is a victory, and every session on the wall is an opportunity to connect with your body in a meaningful way·

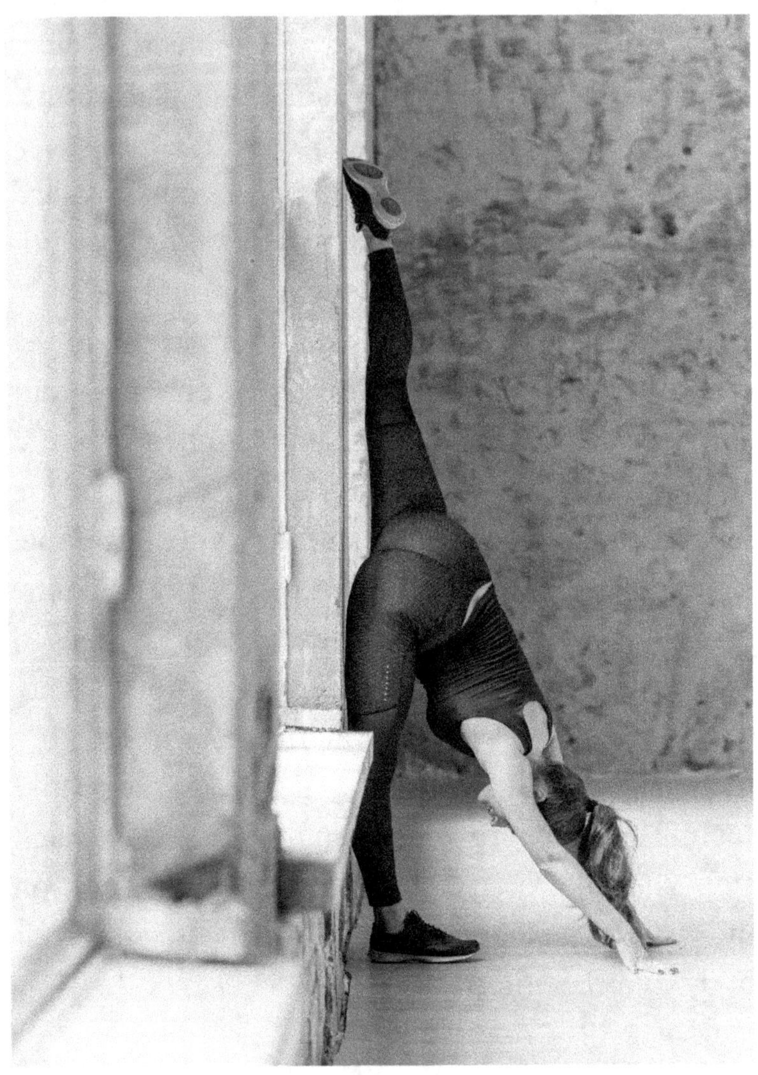

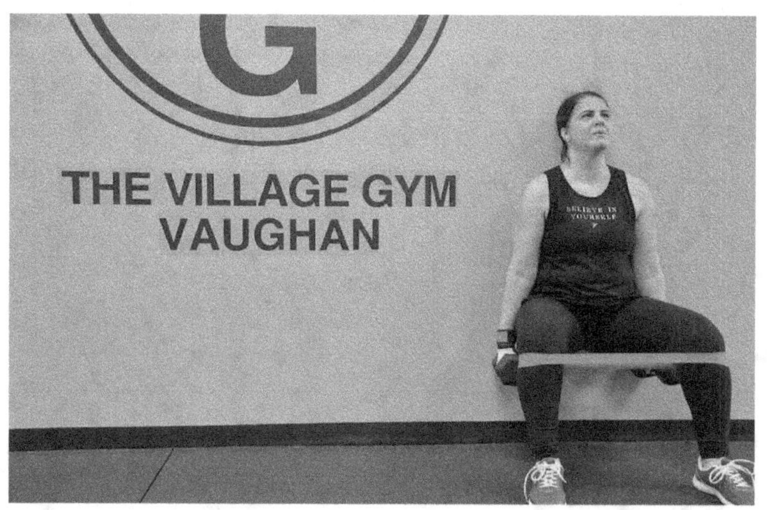
THE VILLAGE GYM
VAUGHAN
BELIEVE IN
YOURSELF

Wall Plate For Seniors Over 60

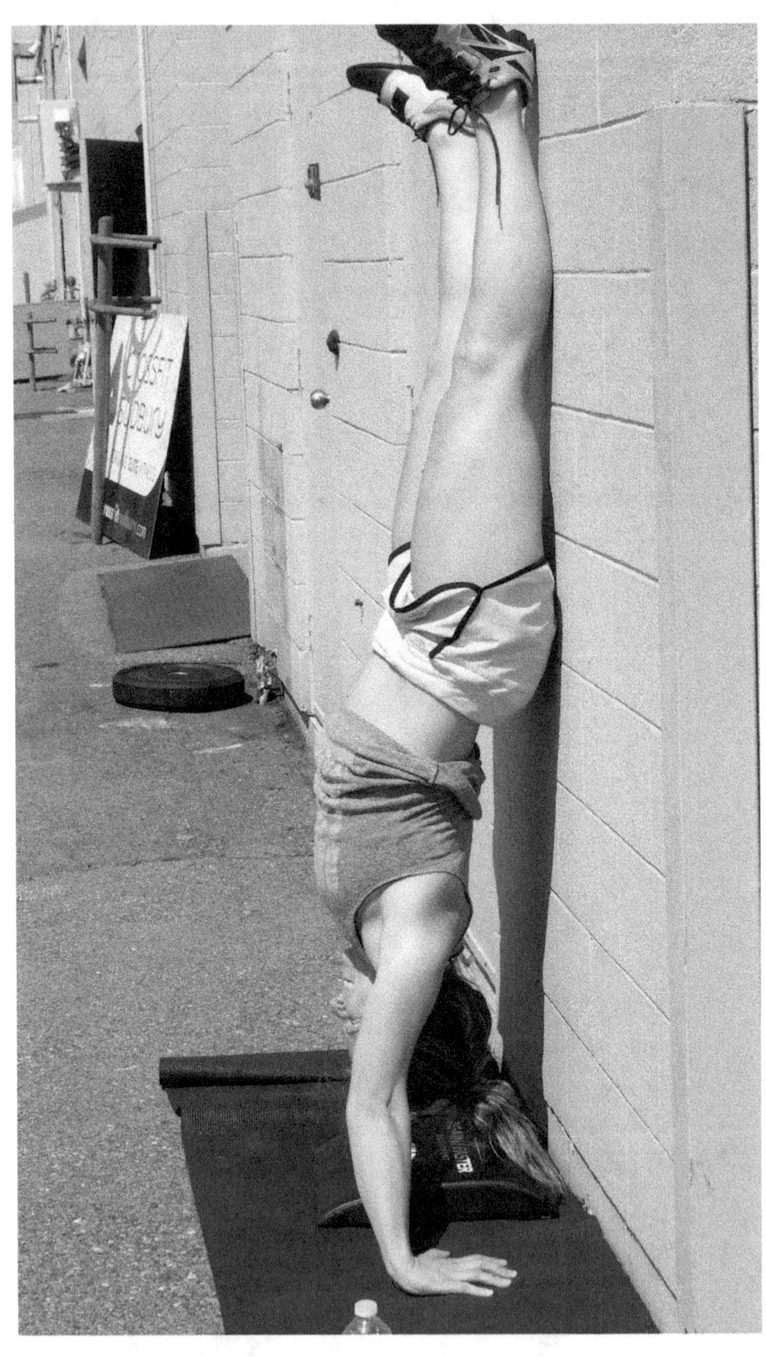

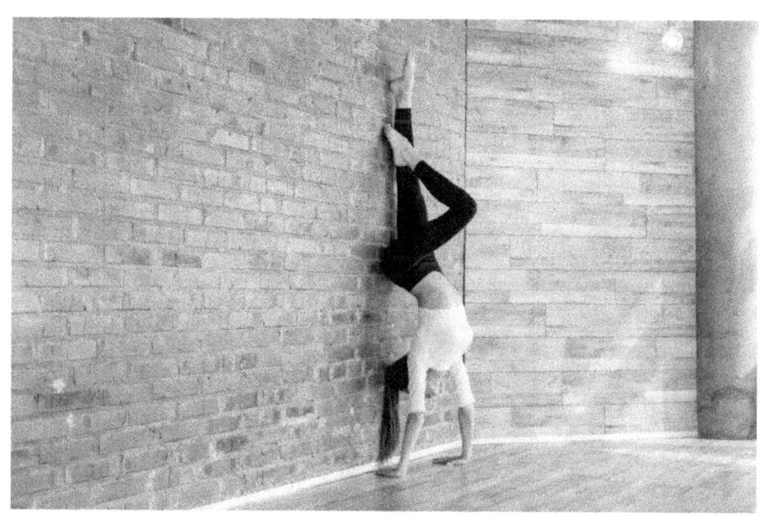

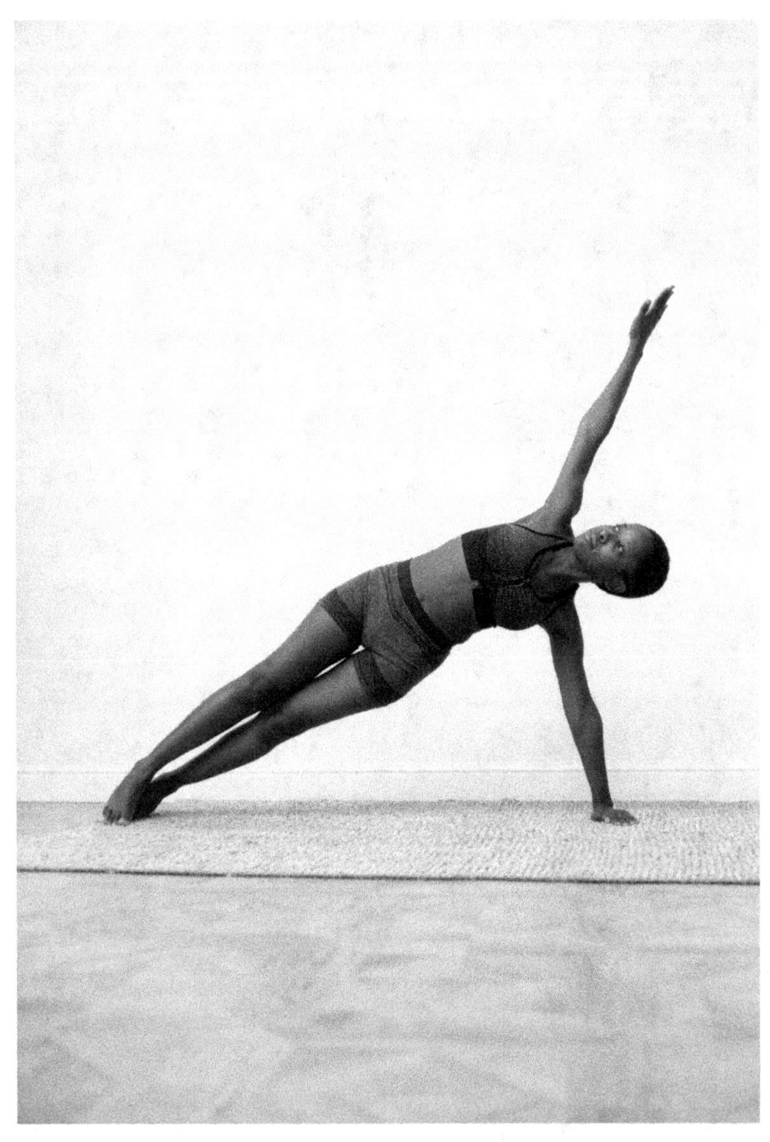